PRACTICAL YOGA

PRACTICAL YOGA

June Johns

in collaboration with

Mehr S. Fardoonji

with photographs by

Jack Smith

DAVID & CHARLES

NEWTON ABBOT · LONDON

VANCOUVER

0 7153 6642 4

Set in 11 on 13pt Bembo
by Avontype (Bristol) Limited
and printed in Great Britain
by Biddles Ltd Guildford
for David & Charles (Holdings) Limited
South Devon House Newton Abbot Devon

Published in Canada by Douglas David &
Charles Limited   3645 McKechnie Drive
West Vancouver BC

Contents

Part One

WHAT IS YOGA?

1 The Meaning of Yoga

Yoga, like St Paul, is all things to all men. To the mystic it is a method of achieving samadhi, or nirvana; to the religious, a path to God; to the aesthete, a means of subduing or controlling the demands of the body to the needs of the mind, and to the majority of Westerners it is an aid to a fuller life.

The word itself is derived from the Sanskrit for 'yoke' and the entire philosophy is aimed at uniting the individual with the universe. Although it is unknown how, where and when Yoga began, its principles have been documented for thousands of years and are common to many ancient cultures as diverse as Egypt, China and India. Buddha himself was a Yogi six centuries before the birth of Christ, and while Yoga has absorbed many ideas and has developed considerably through the centuries, its basic concepts have not changed.

There is good in every person and every thing is the belief; each man will achieve fulfilment and self-realisation if he learns to know himself physically, mentally and spiritually so that he has complete control over himself and his desires.

Yoga is not a religion. It does not claim to be the only path to salvation, nor does it exclude anyone for any reason. Old or young, sick or well, rich or poor, all can practise it, and because no single one of the five main methods of following Yoga could suit everybody, each person is expected initially to select the path most suited to himself.

Perhaps because of the hope it offers, Yoga has succeeded and flourished while so many other philosophies have wilted with time. Yoga requires no one to change his personality, for there is a path to suit everyone. It teaches man never to despair if he falls short of his aim, that worry is bad, for it hinders spiritual progress, and that in any case tomorrow is another day which must begin without one being soured by regrets from today.

Force and fear have no place. Neither body nor mind must be over-strained, and because there are no threats of punishment in a future hell, one is encouraged to look within oneself when anything goes wrong, rather than to blame external causes. In fact, man is taught that if he follows Yoga concepts, he can control his own happiness and his own destiny, but on no account must he try to control that of others.

One of the gems of the *Mahabharata*, the Indian epic which is one of the great religious classics of the world, is the *Bhagavad Gita*. It is to the Hindus what the Sermon on the Mount is to Christians, and it contains an unparalleled summing-up of Yoga. It is a dialogue between the warrior, Arjuna, and his friend, Krishna, who is the incarnation of God. Allegorically the *Gita* depicts the conflict between the two selves which dwells in every human. Arjuna is reluctant to take part in a fratricidal war in which he would be compelled to kill his kinsmen and he asks what he should do. Krishna replies that as Arjuna is a warrior, trained to defend his people, he cannot desert them in their hour of need, no matter how troubled his mind.

'Action alone concerns you,' added Krishna, knowing that of the five main paths of Yoga, the one concerning action was that most suited to his friend. 'Never its fruits. Stability in success or failure, this balance is called Yoga.'

Written nearly 2,500 years ago, these words are not unlike those by Rudyard Kipling in his poem, 'If':

If you can meet with Triumph and Disaster
And treat those two impostors just the same.

Duty in this context means keeping faith with oneself regardless of the consequences. Because much of Yoga sounds easier than in fact it is, and because there is no human failing beyond its scope, there is no condemnation of those who fall by the wayside. Tolerance is all-embracing and even the greatest Yogi would urge the failures to pick themselves up and try again. No one is regarded as infallible and novices are urged never to invest their teachers with 'holiness'. Success or failure, they must be accepted equally.

The way, then, to start Yoga is to follow its directions in getting to know yourself so that you can choose the path most likely to suit your temperament. Yoga has been likened to a cartwheel with many spokes each interlaced with cobwebs. The hub is the goal, self-realisation or being at one with God, depending on your point of view or on your religion. The outer rim is where we all begin, and the basic belief is that all of us, willy-nilly, are working our way towards the centre. Most of us are unaware of our journey or of its goal. We stray from the path, linger for years or perhaps a whole lifetime without regaining it. Yogis are those who are conscious of where they are going and who aim to get there in the shortest possible time.

There are as many individual spokes as there are people in the world, but to help communicate the essentials of Yoga the teachers of old divided the 'spokes' into five principal paths. None is entirely separate from the others; they overlap sometimes two and three together, and of course there are other paths. But the majority of students can recognise readily with a brief study which section he would best fit, according to his temperament and the stage and condition of his life.

Yoga is not, of course, the only philosophy to recognise the need for different courses of training for various temperaments. Indeed, one of the leading schools of thought in the study of temperament

was that of the Austrian philosopher and scientist, Rudolf Steiner (1861–1925). Steiner believed that most people could be divided, roughly into one of four basic categories — melancholic, phlegmatic, sanguine or choleric. In the children's schools where his methods are widely practised, each teacher is taught not only to recognise his own temperament so that he does not make the mistake of trying to impose it on his pupils, but to get to know each child so as to categorise them into the basic type to which they belong. Naturally, two or more characteristics are often present in the same person, but as a rule one predominates.

It is interesting to note that Steiner's categories are similar to those divided by the four major Yoga paths. Broadly speaking, the melancholic could be the sort of person who follows the emotional route of Bhakti; the phlegmatic could follow the intellectual Yoga of Jnana; the sanguine, the all-embracing Raja, and the choleric, the Yoga of action, Karma.

Steiner taught that each temperament has its good and its bad aspect. The melancholic can be depressive to the point of suicide, while on the credit side, he is artistic and creative. The phlegmatic can be lazy and lethargic, but on the other hand he can be dependable and loyal. The sanguine can spread his interests so wide that he becomes like a grasshopper, leaping from one interest to another and seldom finishing anything he starts. But his very breadth of vision enables him to have perspective, to be able to unite warring factions and to remain tolerant. The choleric, at worst, is a domineering bully, but at best he is an able leader. Steiner taught his disciples to recognise the traits and to encourage the good aspects while curbing the bad.

These, then, roughly follow four of the main paths of Yoga, and the fifth, Hatha Yoga, is comparable to the child's attending school in the first place, since most people who take up the study of Yoga begin by practising Hatha.

It must be understood that there is nothing to prevent us from following any one of the Yoga paths, even one least suited to our particular temperament. But only by choosing the one most relevant to our way of life can we expect to be successful. The path is not supposed to be an obstacle-course with difficulties deliberately included; rather it should be the one which seems easiest to follow, and self-honesty in recognising one's own shortcomings and weaknesses is of paramount importance right from the start.

What man is only beginning fully to understand this century, that each and every species depends on the next, that the smallest atom in a grain of sand obeys the same immutable laws that keep the planets on their course, seems to have been grasped by Yogis thousands of years ago. The poet John Donne had an inkling when he wrote, 400 years ago: 'No man is an Island, entire of itself; every man is a piece of the Continent, a part of the main.' And: 'Any man's death diminishes me, because I am involved in Mankind; And therefore never send to know for whom the bell tolls; it tolls for thee.'

Each student of Yoga is taught that his every word and action is capable of influencing other people. What he says today may sow a seed in the son of his friend. Like an echo that goes on and on, or the ripples in water when a pebble is thrown into a lake, the effects could be wide-reaching and endless. Each effect has a cause, each cause an effect, and so Yogis must always be aware of the responsibility they bear.

Since one's journey through life must, to a great extent, depend on one's talents, Yogis are warned of the dangers of setting their sights beyond the range of their abilities. According to Yoga philosophy, it is better to be a good road-sweeper than a bad bank manager and students are exhorted to follow their Svadharama. Loosely translated as 'destiny', Svadharama relates to the age of more static societies than our own when a boy usually followed his father's trade, having been trained from childhood. He did not waste time, thought or energy searching for the right career.

An Indian story illustrates the point. A son spent his life caring for his blind parents. One day on his way from the well with water, he was stopped by a beggar who asked to be fed. The boy told him to wait, that his parents' needs had to be satisfied first. The beggar suddenly transformed himself into Vishnu, the incarnation of God. Still the boy refused, albeit regretfully, to serve him before attending to his parents. And of course Vishnu praised him for not swerving from his duty.

Svadharama, then, is the sense of duty in following one's true vocation, upon which all spiritual progress depends.

2 Hatha Yoga:

The Yoga of Physical Health

Having examined the possible means of approaching Yoga, those interested should bear in mind the advice offered by teachers throughout the ages. They advise students to begin with Hatha Yoga, the control of the body.

To Westerners this is the usual way of learning Yoga and, in fact, many are satisfied with improving their health and do not delve any deeper into the philosophy. Others begin with Hatha and continue along one or more of the other paths. It is entirely a matter of personal choice, and learning Hatha Yoga alone can bring immense improvement and enrichment of everyday life.

One of the main advantages is that being a physical practice, progress is readily apparent and capable of being charted. It is easier for Westerners to understand since philosophy of any kind is less familiar to us than to, say, Hindus.

The word 'Hatha' stems from 'ha' meaning 'sun' and 'tha', 'moon', the former being a positive force and the latter negative, neither being better nor worse than the other, just different and equally essential to life. This philosophy of dualism is not confined to Yoga. It is included in one form or another in most religions, but the Yoga belief is that our body is enlivened by these twin currents, and when both are in complete equilibrium we enjoy perfect health. The Chinese philosophy of Yin and Yang — Yin being the feminine, negative and passive, and Yang being the masculine, positive and creative, holds that their balance sustains and engenders the universe. Similarly the physical science of acupuncture used by the Chinese for thousands of years is based on the belief of there

being certain meridians or paths throughout the body along which these twin currents flow. Ill-health alters the flow, and the insertion and manipulation of needles at strategic points can reverse or otherwise change the balance of the currents, bring them back into equilibrium, and so restore health.

The presence of negative and positive currents coursing through the body is no mere conjecture. Recent neurological research in Britain has shown that we are equipped with two sets of nerves — a fine network which transmits, by means of positive currents, the sensations of pain to the spinal cord and so to the brain; the other, thicker nerves, situated alongside, conduct negative currents. When the thick nerves are stimulated, they can block out the positive currents travelling along the 'pain' nerves. Observe what happens if you bruise yourself. Instinctively you rub the painful spot, thus activating the thick, negative nerves so that their response impedes the pain signals.

It is interesting to note that Buddhism came to China from India and that Buddha himself became a Yogi. He had tried various methods in his search for self-realisation, including some rigorous regimes, but he found none of these extremes successful and he came to embrace the middle way of Yoga.

Although these ideas may sound new to Western ears, they have been accepted and practised in the East for thousands of years. To make them more readily understood, imagine that Ha and Tha are two oxen tied together by the yoke of Yoga. When the two work in harmony, energy is utilised to the full. You, the man, are in complete charge and both obey your directions; if one strains against the other, energy is wasted and stresses occur. The purpose of Hatha Yoga is to let each man have complete control of his own mind and body so that all parts work in unison with minimum effort and maximum gain.

It might be thought that putting such emphasis on the body is selfish, especially when one remembers that many early Christians delighted in mortifying the flesh for the greater glory of God. But Yogis believe that the body is a machine to be looked after and controlled by the will. Imagine beating a car to subdue its noisy engine, giving it inferior petrol, dirty oil or insufficient servicing. It is unlikely that it would take us where we wanted to go without causing us considerable delay and inconvenience. So it is with the body. Only by understanding its needs, controlling its requirements and keeping it in perfect working order can we rely on it to do what we want, when we want it to. Then, when we set out on a course of action — whether sleeping, working or enjoying ourselves — we can afford to forget the body knowing that it will not let us down.

Anyone who has had an illness, or even a headache, can appreciate the lack of concentration and sometimes the inability to rest or work caused by physical pain or discomfort. The Yoga way to be healthy is not just for the pleasure of good health, but to release the mind and spirit so that they can be concerned with other things without being hampered by an inefficient, obtrusive body.

Because the control of the body is only a means to achieve absolute control of the mind, that is, the brain and the emotions, it might be argued that a more direct method of controlling the mind by concentration or meditation could be preferable. In general, however, this is not so. If you think of the mind and the body as two express trains racing each other on parallel lines, you will see that should the body train slow down and begin to stop, for a little while the other train — the mind — might continue at the same speed, but very soon it too will begin to slow down and will eventually stop.

So it is with us. If we can still the body — and to most people this is much easier than trying to control something as amorphous and undisciplined as the average mind — it usually follows that the latter can be trained to obey.

Those who have ever been seriously worried will recall how the mind tends to behave like a rat in a trap — it frets and fumes, it races round in circles covering the same ground in search of an escape route which is not there. By using the very practical techniques of Hatha Yoga and Pranayama (the Yogic method of absorbing vitality by correct breathing) the emotions can be returned to balance and reason restored. This is not, of course, achieved overnight but as the limbs and muscles, stiff from disuse, gradually begin to respond to the regular exercises, so the mind and emotions react to the discipline imposed upon them, to the advantage of the whole body.

It is quite possible that others will prefer to attempt self-control and self-realisation by tackling the mind before the body. Hatha Yoga is not for them. But for most of us it is the easiest path, and the one with which this book is chiefly concerned.

To begin with, we must become aware of our body and its organs. Any animal has a more instinctive understanding of its own body than we have. Watch a cat waken and stretch itself, muscle by muscle, limb by limb, before moving into action. Watch a puppy drop in its tracks the moment it is exhausted and sleep, utterly relaxed until it has, so to speak, recharged its batteries. Civilisation has, unfortunately, brought us very far from our animal origins and we would do well to remember that physically at least, we are not so very different from other living creatures and we deny our heritage at our peril. Ideally we should emulate other animals: eat only when hungry, drink only when thirsty and rest only when tired instead of organising our daily round by the demands of society and the clock.

Because Yogis have never denied their affinity, if not their direct relationship, with animals, many of the exercises developed through the centuries have been given the names of animals: the Dog, the Fish, the Cow, the Locust, to name but a few. Perhaps primitive man, like his near relations, automatically used the muscles which we now have to re-train before they can fully serve us in the ways nature intended.

THE SPINE

The first part of the body to be considered is also the most important, the spine. Yogis are taught that a man is as old or as young as his spine is supple, and it is the pivot of nearly every Yoga exercise and pose. It is a fact well-known by actors that when a young man has to play the part of an old, he bends his back and walks stiffly, as, in fact, so many old people walk. But they need not. It is through lack of movement that the spine becomes stiff and the discs of gristle between the vertebrae become worn and compressed so further restricting movement. A vicious circle is created. It is no myth that people shrink as they grow older, but the shrinkage can actually be reversed by the practice of Hatha Yoga exercises. Students are advised to measure their height before beginning Yoga, and again at frequent intervals. It is common for people of all ages to increase their height by inches within months of daily exercises, as the spine is strengthened and can so support the body without being compressed, vertebra against vertebra.

The importance of the spine is known to all, for an injury to the column affects the whole body while a flexible spine radiates vitality. The theory in Hatha Yoga is that the negative pole of the body is situated in the coccyx, the lowest vertebra, that the positive pole is at the top of the skull, and that the tension maintained between them is the life force carried along the spinal cord. From the base, the force called the Kundalini — the 'coiled one' — can be drawn up to each of the seven centres — 'Chakras' — situated in the spine, to produce consciousnesses unknown to ordinary men, such as

telepathy, clairvoyance, extra-sensory perception and various occult faculties. Understandably such powers are developed only by experienced and dedicated Yogis. Yoga teachers explain that once one has achieved these faculties, there is a great temptation to remain at this stage and capitalise on the powers acquired. But by abusing or prostituting them, a Yogi can destroy himself. Instead one should proceed further until the life force, or Kundalini, reaches the top of the skull and one achieves Samadhi, or self-realisation.

To digress, I met a Yogi some years ago who had reached an advanced stage in the art and he demonstrated how he could stop his flow of blood. He took a steel knitting-needle, allowed both it and his right cheek to be examined and then he stuck the needle from the inside of his mouth until it protruded outside his cheek. He then allowed it to be pulled out. At no time did one drop of blood appear, nor did he flinch or show signs of discomfort, and when the needle was removed it was impossible to find the exact spot at which it had penetrated. During the operation, which lasted two or three minutes, no sign of a pulse could be found on the Yogi, although it began to beat strongly and evenly when his demonstration ended. Even those who do not achieve the ultimate invariably develop a clearer mind and greater health.

PRANA

Another basic concept of Hatha Yoga is the necessity for increasing our daily intake of Prana. It is derived from the Sanskrit meaning 'absolute energy' and it is believed to be *in* the air, but it is not air; to be *in* water, but it is not water, and so on with all the basic necessities of life — food, sunshine, sleep. Unless we know how best to acquire Prana in sufficient quantities, and having acquired it, how to store it within us, it is unlikely that we can achieve the mental and physical health aimed at by Hatha Yoga.

One of the main ways of taking in Prana is by breathing correctly — Pranayama. Considering that man can exist for only a few minutes without breathing, it is astounding how few of us know how to do it correctly. What is realised instinctively by every animal seems to elude modern man. Most of us use less than one-fifth of our lung capacity and so constantly have an excess of impurities passing through our bloodstream, impurities which impair the digestion and poison the system and which could be removed automatically by a sufficient intake of oxygen.

People who, on account of frailty or disease, are unable to follow Hatha Yoga exercises, will benefit immeasurably simply by following Pranayama (see Chapter 10). Indian philosophers say that man is born with just so many breaths in his body, implying that those who breathe quickly, die sooner. This is comparable to the belief of some modern zoologists that the lifespan of an animal is determined by its pulse rate, that those with slow rates within the species have greater longevity than those with fast. Whether or not either of these theories is valid, anyone who practises Yogic breathing exercises will, within the space of a few weeks, be able to slow down his pulse rate at will.

RELAXATION

Directly related to Pranayama is the Hatha Yoga third concept that no organism can work effectively unless it can relax completely at will. In fact, most Westerners who seek to learn Yoga do so because of their inability to relax without the aid of drugs. It is probable that the tensions created in our bodies, if not our minds, could be removed if we had enough physical exercise each day. Usually, however, we not only lack the exercise, but we are also unable to locate the exact seat of our tensions — the Yoga method of relaxation teaches us how to identify and deal with each one. Once acquired, it is a knack which renders sleeping pills and tranquillisers unnecessary.

Many who embark on the purely physical aspects of Yoga are sceptical about many of the ideas and the beliefs, as indeed were the authors. Is there such a thing as Prana? Are there really negative and positive currents flowing through our spines? But if there is no harm in going along with the theories, why not try them? Many of the old wives' tales of long ago were scorned by modern man until now when scientists are constantly discovering not only that the homely remedies worked, but that they obeyed scientific laws. It seems that we are reluctant to accept facts for which we are offered no proof. But it is worthwhile to remember that some of the most sceptical beginners of Hatha Yoga have become so impressed with the proof of their own improved health, vitality and concentration, that they have decided not to stop with the physical exercises, but to embrace a second or even third form of Yoga.

superimposed over your present dislike of the person. It is not an easy exercise. To most of us who, in some perverse way, enjoy disliking someone, it is very difficult but it can be done and with practice it becomes more easy — and it works. We not only learn compassion and understanding, but also discrimination and Yama becomes easier.

All people have a portion of good in them and perhaps it is our own short-sightedness that makes us unaware of it. There are sound practical reasons for the advisability of channelling our feelings of hatred into less-destructive emotions. Psychologically it is harmful to repress feelings of aggression, but since civilisation decrees that we must try to live at peace with our neighbours, we can best avoid blood-pressure, stomach ulcers and other manifestations of bottled-up hatred by substituting another, more acceptable emotion, namely one of understanding and of seeing good in those to whom we are not particularly attracted.

The emotions most likely to impede Yama are:
greed
anger
non-discrimination
lust
pride
jealousy

The best way to combat these passions is to replace them with their positive aspects. Take greed, for example. Supposing someone has an object which you covet. You might ask yourself why you should not steal it since the owner has less need or appreciation of it than you. A Christian might answer, 'because stealing is a sin', or 'because it is written in the Gospel that thou shalt not steal or covet'. The Asiatic, according to the Hindu philosophy, will answer that you hurt no one more than yourself when you steal, for a bad conscience causes fear, fear causes toxins to flow from the glands into the bloodstream, and toxins poison the body, therefore in the long run the thief poisons himself by his own actions. A theft, says Karma Yoga, is always the intrusion of the ego into a foreign sphere

of will: in fact you impose your will upon someone else if only by depriving them of their possession. It adds that our attachment to material objects is the result of egoistic activity and that a man who wishes to make spiritual progress will not want to fetter himself with his acquisitions. Rather like Henry David Thoreau who believed that true freedom belonged only to the man who had no possessions, a belief also propounded by Christ and His disciples, the Karma Yogi believes that material possessions act as fetters which deter all spiritual progress.

The conducts towards oneself — Niyama — are:
cleanliness or purity–Soucha
contentment–Santosha
austerity–Tapas
study–Svadhyaya
devotion–Ishvara or Pranidhrana
moderation in sex–Brahmacharya

Most of these precepts are self-evident, but contentment must not be confused with complacency. It is rather tranquillity, the ability to control desires so as not to quest after the unattainable. Study increases knowledge of self and of the particular Yoga path being followed, and devotion can be to whatever God the student worships, or else to the ideals of Yoga.

The parable told to illustrate the essence of Karma Yoga — that work is just another form of worship — is of an extremely devout Yogi who spent most of his life praying to Vishnu. One day the Yogi, Narada, was visited by Vishnu, the incarnation of God, who told him that although he had done quite well, he would make better progress if he tried harder. Narada was both mortified and a little indignant. He could not see where he had fallen short and he had difficulty knowing how he could improve himself. Seeing his dilemma, Vishnu told him to go to the next village to watch a peasant who, said Vishnu, was a greater Yogi than Narada.

Together Vishnu and Narada walked to the next village where they silently observed the peasant all day. He rose early, ate a meagre breakfast, said a brief prayer and then spent the rest of the day working in the fields. At evening he returned home, prepared and ate his meal, said another brief prayer and went to bed. Narada asked what was so wonderful about this, adding that he devoted many more hours of each day to worship while the peasant's prayers were minimal. Vishnu sighed. Obviously Narada had not understood.

'I want you to take these two buckets,' he said. 'Fill them to the very brim with water and carry them to the other end of the village and back again to me without spilling one drop.'

It was a long, straggling village and Narada had great difficulty ensuring that not one drop was spilt. At length he returned triumphant, his mission accomplished.

'Now,' asked Vishnu, 'How often did you think of me while you were fulfilling this task?'

Narada protested that it had required all his concentration to keep his balance and avoid spilling the water, and that he had had no time to think of God or prayer.

'Exactly,' replied Vishnu. 'Now you can understand the peasant. He was doing the work for which he was destined, my work, and it took all his time and energy, leaving little in which he could sit and pray. For work, also, is a form of worship.'

There is often the question of whether work is done for the doer or for the recipient. In Karma Yoga there is no difference — work is regarded as a form of enlightened self-interest. It satisfies both self and others, and the Karma Yogi must never imagine that he is doing the world a great service or that he can revolutionise mankind. Reforming the world is compared to straightening the curly tail of a dog. If you take hold of the tip and stretch it out, it will remain straight. But the instant it is released it will spring back into its original position. And so with life. While you weed one patch of land, more weeds will be springing up elsewhere; put right one wrong and often another wrong will be set into motion, perhaps not to be apparent for years.

Examples of this inexorable chain-reaction may be seen in the great campaigns and successive legislation of the past; for example, the repeal of slavery produced many homeless people who had no one to feed them and they drifted to the ghettoes of the city slums of America. The recent abortion laws of Britain which, while just and necessary, led to numerous abuses, each needing correction.

The belief in cause and effect, of retributive justice inherent in Karma Yoga extends to the chain of reincarnation. Whereas the Christian belief is of an after-life in heaven or hell, the Hindu Yoga belief is that we reap what we sow by returning to earth as someone, or something, else. This rebirth theory spread from India to Europe and was taught by Pythagoras in about 580 BC and later spread to Japan as part of Buddhist doctrine. It is not fully accepted by Westerners, many believing it is allegorical, explaining the immutable laws of Karma, of cause and effect.

In essence Karma is a practical philosophy dictating that one should live in the present moment, undeterred by the worries of yesterday or the fears of tomorrow, giving oneself fully to the work at hand. Easterners crystallise it in their saying, 'All creative beings are owners of their works, heirs of their works, children and slaves of their works.' The Christian equivalent would be, 'By their fruits shall ye know them.'

4 Bhakti Yoga:
The Yoga of Love or Devotion

The two main ways of comprehending the world are by feeling and by reason: the former is known as Bhakti Yoga. Because it is available to everyone, rich or poor, sick or well, and because we are born with the instinct to love, it appears to be the easiest path. This is not so. While it is easy to love someone dear to us, things which are beautiful and people who love us, it can be incredibly difficult to lavish those same affections on objects and people which do not appeal to us.

The love demanded of the Bhakti must be all-embracing and unquestioning. There must be neither expectation nor hope of its being returned and it must conquer — or kill — both pride and the ego. It is the sort of love given by a mother to her child. She does not abandon him when he says he hates her and that he wishes she would die, nor does she put her own comfort first when he needs her. She does not hesitate to chastise him for his own good, even when she would prefer to indulge him. When he grows up and marries, she may be sad to lose him, but happy because of his happiness; and so with the Yogi who accepts either success or failure with equanimity.

But while this willing sacrifice of self is comparatively easy for a loving mother, the Bhakti Yogi must give exactly the same quality and quantity of devotion, first to the rest of his family, then to his friends and neighbours through to his enemies and adversaries, and before anyone embarks on the Bhakti path he is advised to look within himself to see if he has the capacity for such selflessness. Some introverts, in particular, might find difficulties and would do well to consider another form of Yoga.

Because the philosophy of Yoga is to make the chosen path as easy as possible, the Bhakti is advised to begin his devotions with an object — or person — rather than with an abstract idea. Most of us have more difficulty in grasping a concept than in understanding something visual. The child can readily accept the theory of heat-expanding metals when his teacher has demonstrated it by passing a metal ball through a ring, then by trying to pass it through the same ring when the ball has been heated and has expanded. The theory of gravity demonstrated by Newton's apple, the steam power by Watt's kettle: there are numerous tangible examples which parallel the Yoga teaching that God, or the cosmic force, resides in every thing and every person on earth, there for us to see and to worship.

Religions of all kinds have recognised the human need to see a representation of God. Christian statues, icons, crosses, tribal totem poles, Asiatic cow or snake worship all derive from this basic need. The Bhakti, therefore, selects his chosen object. He must not disclose it to anyone, even — in the event of its being a person — to that person. If he were to do so he might make life unnecessarily difficult for himself. The person might ridicule him or become resentful, and in the beginning at least, the Bhakti should try to avoid meeting his own ego head-on. The object of his choice is but a tool to teach him how to love and how to search for the good in all things. It is not to be loved just for itself and for its own qualities, but also for its being related to everything else in the universe. The Yogi studies it with his heart and with his mind, seeking out its best points and discovering for himself the similarities it has with other things and other people. He relates it to the scheme of things and no matter how irritating some aspects might be — perhaps in a tree that won't bloom or in a person who behaves badly — he must find out enough good to eclipse the bad aspects.

It is not only into the objects themselves that he pours his love; his thoughts, words and deeds must be coloured by it. The platitude, 'it's the thought that counts' becomes true for the Bhakti, and he must realise how different the outcome of his smallest action might be if it is done without love. He must put all of himself into his work, again with no yearning for a successful result.

The belief that love attracts love is shown in the orthodox Hindu marriage ceremony when the father of the bride has to kneel before the bride-groom and touch his feet — a formal gesture usually reserved for juniors to perform towards their seniors. The father of the bride is ritually recognising the God in his son-in-law. To whom else would a father give his child?

Many people perform their duties in this way. Nurses who, by loving their patients or their work, are able to perform tasks which would otherwise be repulsive, and their attitude of willingness and love in turn helps their patients. Similarly a teacher who loves both her subject and her pupils is usually a great deal more effective than one who cares for neither. The Bhakti trains himself to approach good and evil with equal welcome and to accept that although the presence of love is often barely detectable, it will enhance everything and everyone it touches.

There is an Indian tale of the arrival of the Parsees when they fled from the Islamic invasion of Persia in the eighth century AD. When they landed on the shores of India, their leader approached the resident rajah and asked if his people might settle in the region, but it was a densely populated area and regretfully the rajah refused, demonstrating how crowded his people were by presenting the Parsee with a glass filled to the brim with milk. One drop more, he explained, and it would over-flow. The Parsee took a pinch of sugar and dropped it in the glass. Invisible, it did not cause the milk to overflow but in a small way it sweetened it as, he insisted, would his people if they were permitted to settle in India. And so they came to stay. Bhakti is like the sugar in the milk of life; it sweetens it. The Bhakti is taught to seek out the good in evil by accepting that both qualities are usually present in all things and all deeds. Fire burns but it also warms and comforts; a man may drown in water but it quenches thirst and sustains life.

There are two ways of seeing goodness in all things: the first is by recognising it in the presence of great things — mountains, the sky, the wind and the sea; and then progressing to the small, the insignificant, the grain of sand. This is the progression from the gross to the subtle. The second way is by recognising good in things and people beloved, and progressing to seek it out in its more complicated form, in the apparently unlovable. This is progressing from the simple to the complex.

The mother, for example, can begin with her own child and then go on to give her love to its friends. When the child grows up she must embrace the marriage partner. She must not restrict her love to those she likes. Whenever she finds resentment and antipathy arising she must not turn aside but rather pause to envelop the ill-feelings with good-will, using her love as a lever to conquer her ego.

It is a human failing to keep the focus of love narrow, but just as newly weds who are so wrapped up in each other that they have no time for others eventually have to widen their circle if the marriage is to succeed, so must the Bhakti, his ultimate goal being when he can merge himself with the object of his love so that the two become indivisible, both being parts of the cosmos.

The parable illustrating the Bhakti Yogi is of a rather stupid pupil who so worshipped his guru that he sat spellbound and never thought to ask questions like the other students. He hung on to every word and spent his free time thinking of him and repeating his name. One day the student went for a walk along the riverbank, repeating his guru's name incessantly. He was so absorbed that he failed to notice that the river curved and he walked right into it. But he did not sink. To the astonishment of nearby villagers, he walked right across the water. They hurried to tell the guru, emphasising that his name must have tremendous power if so dull a student could walk on water by repeating it. The guru was surprised, but not so much as they. He had always had a good opinion of himself and he believed he was superior to most men. He set off for the river and, repeating his own name, walked into it. He sank immediately.

It is a humbling tale, not unlike that in the Bible where the wedding guests who positioned themselves in the best rooms were humiliated and those who went into the lowly rooms were elevated. It illustrates that only the quality of a man's love matters, not his intellect nor his station in life, and that his aim must be to link all men and all things by his love for them and for life itself.

Most sophisticated people despise peasants. In Britain it is a derogatory term, but Yoga makes no distinction between the educated and the ignorant, both being of equal importance. Manual work is not to be despised. In fact any task performed with love ennobles the worker and his work. In the *Gita*, Krishna counsels his friend Arjuna to welcome manual tasks as a means of growing closer to those for whom he does them. He explains that he, Krishna, grooms and feeds his own horse which in return loves him. Everything must be done wholeheartedly; superficial tasks and involvements are best avoided.

Naturally one cannot become a perfect Bhakti immediately, and it is recognised that there are three main stages in his development. First he is the interested Bhakti, who prays to God for a particular thing. He is not to be despised for his humility and for his simple faith, for this too has power. Second there is the disinterested Bhakti who, instead of asking God for material things, either throws himself on God's mercy, seeks wisdom and knowledge as an explorer or inventor, or looks for the purpose and meaning in life while devoting himself to helping society. Lastly there is the perfect Bhakti who sees God in everything, as epitomised in the *Gita* as being

without hatred for any being, friendly, compassionate, without possessiveness, without egoism, equal in pain and pleasure, forgiving, contented. . .

He from whom the world does not shudder away, and who does not shudder away from the world, and who is free from the uprushing of sensuous enthusiasm, anger and fear. . .

He who is not looking for something [for his pleasure or happiness], who is pure, industrious, impartial, untroubled [by what happens]. . .

He who does not exult, is not hostile, does not grieve, does not long [for anything]. . .

The same to foe and friend, and likewise when respected or disrespected, and the same in cold and heat and pleasure and pain, free from attachments, equal when reproached or praised, silent, contented with whatever is. . .

It is a formidable assignment, but those who choose to practise Bhakti Yoga greatly increase their opportunities for happiness. The progress of the Bhakti is from seeing good in the small and familiar and expanding to the universal. God or goodness — the terms are synonymous. Seeing God in small things is not fragmenting Him like pieces of a jigsaw puzzle. The Bhakti sees Him complete though in miniature in each and every thing.

Image-worship, therefore, is the art of experiencing the whole universe within a small visible object so that the worship of an image is not for itself alone but for the God it represents as a part of the cosmos. It is wrong, then, to despise the use of images in worship.

The Bhakti uses all his senses in his search for goodness and self-realisation. The Jnana Yogi, on the other hand, directs his search within himself, stilling his senses and using his intellect, outwardly detached but inwardly intensely concerned. Both, of course, are equally valid methods, but the Bhakti method of applying the senses is recommended for the vast majority of people. The difference between the two has been likened to two sons, the one clinging and dependent, the other independent and leading a separate life. The mother loves them equally and to her they are both as important.

5 Jnana Yoga:

The Yoga of Knowledge or Discrimination

Although this form of Yoga is traditionally that chosen by the intellectual, it is by no means exclusive to the well-educated. In fact because its adherents must develop the ability to think clearly, profoundly and with great moral courage, formal education as we know it in the Western world can be a positive hindrance.

Jnana Yoga accepts that there are two main ways of knowing: that of reading, observing, listening — external influences which add up to cumulative knowledge. The other: innate, true wisdom, being intuitive knowledge. The former is, of course, important but it is the latter which the Jnana Yogi seeks to discover and develop. Thus it is an inward-looking philosophy.

The traditional Indian Yogi often followed this path, forsaking the world to live a spartan existence in order to subjugate the demands of the body to leave his mind free to contemplate the problems of the universe. Even today there are many such men who, while living apart from society, acquire incorruptible wisdom and so are consulted by troubled petitioners who have come to rely on their integrity, their understanding and their assessments.

Before the Jnana Yogi can achieve understanding of man and his place in the universe, he must first gain true understanding of himself and of his mental processes and absolute control of both his body and his mind. He must renounce all superfluous mental and physical activities, the better to concentrate his energies on gaining insight.

Jnana Yoga is called the Yoga of discrimination because at each turn its adherent must decide between right and wrong, importance and trivia, honesty and falsehood, virtue and vice, and have the moral strength to act on his judgement. He seeks to find his own depths before he turns his attention to life, in fact, he follows the ancient Greek advice inscribed at Delphi — 'Know Thyself'.

The Jnana Yogi could play a large part in society given the opportunity. Such dilemmas now facing us as whether or not to develop test-tube babies, whether to reconsider the rectitude of keeping alive by artificial resuscitation patients who can never recover, whether to continue making atomic weapons — all these questions might safely rest in the hands of men of supreme integrity whereas most of us would hesitate to accept unreservedly the advice of politicians, doctors or scientists.

There are two major ways of arriving at the truth: the affirmative, or synthesis, of linking oneself with all creation as the Bhakti does with his love, and the negative process of analysing and eliminating. It is the latter which is used by the Jnana Yogi.

He begins by examining the tools of his consciousness, his senses. For instance, he may consider his eyes, and ask himself, 'Am I my eyes?' He shuts off his other senses and tries to experience fully his sight with as much attention as he can muster. He examines large and small objects in detail, then he closes his eyes. He might even blindfold himself to experience what it would be like if he were blind. But he is still alive, he is stimulated by messages received by his other senses and so he answers, 'No, I am not my eyes.'

He repeats this procedure with each of his other senses, his hearing, his taste, smell and touch, with the same result. By eliminating each one he arrives at the core of his being, the essence of life common to all creatures and, according to Yoga doctrine, inherent in every object, animate or inanimate in the universe.

To achieve the one-pointedness, the intense focus of all his senses upon the one being investigated, the Jnana Yogi half-closes his eyes, except, of course, when his sense of sight is being studied. If he closed his eyes his mind's eye might be invaded with extraneous images. If they were fully open they would be receiving stimuli from his surroundings. By half-closing them he is deliberately shutting out his surroundings while depriving his mind of inward vision. He is, in fact, limiting his focus, restricting his imagination so as to direct his attention to the matter under concentration.

Parallel with his examination of his senses, the Jnana Yogi learns that true freedom cannot be achieved without certain restrictions. As with the Hatha Yogi, he loses his freedom to concentrate if he allows his body to cause him pain and so to interrupt his thoughts. As with the Karma Yogi, he loses his equilibrium and his peace of mind if he allows himself to be over-elated or depressed.

The Jnana Yogi must first decide what it is that he wants to be free to do, a decision contingent upon his complete understanding of himself and of his own nature. He restricts himself in three areas so as to reach the freedom he wants: towards his body, towards the society in which he lives, and towards the universe.

The first of these restrictions is Tapas, which means 'penance', and is performed by keeping the body in a fit state to enable it to function as a tool of the mind. By following the principles of Hatha Yoga he learns to master his appetites and not to be ruled by them. Fasting plays a part, and the self-denial of unnecessary food.

The second, Dana, or the giving of self, is the duty he owes to society. This is interpreted as that due to his parents and friends for all they have done for him, to his family and to the state. He must not believe that the world owes him a living, but on the contrary accepts that he is in debt for all that he has received.

Lastly, Yajna, sacrifice, is the putting back into the world a part of what he has taken from it. As we now realise, just by being alive each person depletes and pollutes the world, and as good farmers sustain their land by enriching it with manure to compensate for their crops, so the Jnana Yogi gives something back in repayment for what he has received. It is with this in mind that the Jnana Yogi must respect all living things.

It would appear that these duties are for the benefit of mankind, as indeed they are, but they are also the means by which the Jnana Yogi makes great spiritual progress. Following the basic Yoga belief that human development is in the direction of the divine or cosmic whole, that man throughout the ages has striven to improve himself and to approach this unity, he is taught to regard his body as a garment and not a part of his real self. By separating the two he avoids the fear of old age or infirmity. He knows that although his body might be imprisoned, or tortured, his inner self cannot be tyrannised or harmed. It can neither be corrupted nor destroyed.

On analysing himself the Jnana Yogi finds that his spiritual development depends on his using his will. To some extent will-development approximates current psychological theory that the infant is more animal than human, that he has no conceptual thought but regards himself almost in the third person. Listen to a child of three demand something. He does not say, 'I want', but, 'Johnny wants'.

A little later the infant develops the ego-will. He sees himself as 'I'. His infant, body-will was that of self-preservation, possessed by all animals and probably located in the old brain, the cerebellum, as against the modern, larger cerebrum. The ego-will is the mind-will, the motor which drives humans. Although this will can be imposed on other people or upon his environment, as when a man gains at the expense of others, the Jnana Yogi learns that misuse creates fetters which retard his progress. By such means he perpetuates suffering, for the Jnana Yogi believes that all sorrow is prevented wish-fulfilment. For example, if a man is accustomed to gratifying his desires, he is likely to be unhappy when thwarted, therefore the more he can control his wish for selfish gratification — by means of his ego-will — the sooner will he be free from unhappiness.

Because of the self-confidence that is acquired with self-control and knowledge, the Jnana Yogi is warned against becoming arrogant, and he must develop the compassion inherent in the practice of Bhakti Yoga. But as he achieves clarity of thought and can often crystallise amorphous problems and see clearly the outcome of a certain course of action, he must not attempt to impose his decisions on other people. There must be no 'I told you so' satisfaction. When asked for advice he is obliged to give it, and then to detach himself.

It follows that a Jnana Yogi is required to set strict limits on his way of life and even his choice of profession. He must not squander his energies on unnecessary activities. He must not use his mind to engage in small-talk or gossip, nor must he proffer advice without being asked for it. His thoughts must be concentrated on his search for the ultimate, and all other mental exercises must be ruthlessly elimated.

His life consists of self-study, the removal of fetters caused by acquisition of power or material goods, and the objectivity not only to seek out, but to find the good in all men and all things. The greater the Jnana Yogi's progress and the nearer he approaches the hub of the wheel of Yoga, the more readily he can penetrate beyond the duality of good and bad and reach the ultimate when he and the universe are at one. The freedom he seeks is not in a place, or in time, but within himself.

The classic story illustrating the Jnana Yogi's search for the cosmic is of two birds who lived in one tree. Right at the top was a beautiful, calm bird which sat silently enjoying the sun. In the lower branches was a restless bird of duller plumage. He hopped this way and that, taking a bite out of all that he saw, and often tasting bitter fruits which caused him pain. Each time he would look up at his remote companion and wish with all his heart to be like him. Each time this happened he found himself able to hop a little higher up the tree.

Unfortunately the wayward bird was prone to follow his appetites and, forgetting his resolutions, would again and again taste the bitter fruits. But each time he strengthened his determination and, gazing up at the golden bird, would try even harder to mend his ways. Presently he controlled his whims and one day found himself on the same branch at the top of the tree. There the bird found that there was no other — it had been a reflection of his inner, perfect self.

Finally, it must be emphasised that although the Jnana Yogi tends to cut himself off from much of the normal intercourse of society, he is not a hermit; he does not reject society. His influence can be strong and pervasive, the more so for being unbiased. His understanding of man can be profound and if society as a whole could call upon a council of such men, possibly the whole of humanity would benefit.

6 Raja Yoga:
The Royal Path

While it is possible, and more than likely, that many people follow Yoga without being aware of it, those who choose Raja Yoga must be subject to a precise discipline to which their whole life must be subservient. Nevertheless the followers will find that to adhere to Raja Yoga they must incorporate much of Hatha, Karma, Bhakti and Jnana. Yoga in itself can be compared to a loaf of bread. It contains flour, water, yeast and salt. Any one of these ingredients eaten alone would not constitute, nor would it taste like, a loaf. Yet incorporated they are unmistakable, and each is an intrinsic, necessary part.

Imagine following Hatha Yoga without incorporating the detachment inherent in Karma; one might become obsessed with the competitive spirit and might even harm oneself in attempting poses too difficult for an ill-prepared body. Consider Karma Yoga without embracing Bhakti to provide the love necessary to perform all work well, or Jnana to provide the knowledge to discriminate between worthy and unworthy aims. And the Bhakti must, of necessity, practise sufficient Hatha to keep his body fit and enough Karma to provide the detachment which ensures that he will not be downcast when the object of his devotion does not reciprocate his love. The Jnana Yogi cannot be effective without the compassion of Bhakti to ensure humility, the Karma to ensure tenacity of purpose, and the Hatha to enable his mind to control his body.

Thus the nearer the hub of the wheel approaches, the closer become the separate spokes, overlapping and intermingling, and Raja Yoga is a combination of all the paths. By Hatha we eliminate the obstacles which our body might put in the way of self-realisation. By Karma we purify our actions and achieve detachment from the results. By Bhakti we intensify the power of love, and by Jnana we find that knowledge and real freedom is within us.

Practically, Raja Yoga consists of eight progressive steps, known as the limbs, which must be strictly followed in their correct order as if they were rungs of a ladder. Each must be fully mastered before the next can be attempted.

They are:

1 Yama–conduct towards others
2 Niyama–conduct towards oneself
3 Asana–the physical postures of Hatha Yoga
4 Pranayama–breath control
5 Pratyahara–discipline of the senses
6 Dharana–concentration
7 Dhyana–meditation
8 Samadhi–self-realisation

1 Yama, referred to in Chapter 3, teaches that we must cause neither harm nor pain to any other being. While we must be willing to help one and all, we must not aid or abet in the commission of crime or sins, but, as if we were a train travelling on fixed rails to a certain goal, we must be available for all who wish to use us, so long as we are not deflected from our route. Its six observances are:

(a) Ahimsa: non-injury and non-violence. If you believe that everything has a central core of goodness, then you must refrain from damaging all things. In practice it means that a Raja Yogi must be a vegetarian to avoid killing animals, and a pacifist so as not to kill other men, no matter where his temporal or civic duties may appear to lie. He must not use corporal punishment nor must he kill by such remote means as insecticides and germ warfare. There can be no exceptions. A Raja Yoga has dedicated his life to his beliefs and he must be prepared to stand by them.

(b) Satya: truthfulness. In itself, honesty is not enough. For the Raja Yogi it must be allied with consideration for others, so that although his thoughts and words must always conform to the facts, people must not be told what would hurt them, what would be cruel to them, even though it were the truth. The great Yogi Ramakrishna put it that true spirituality was in making the heart and the lips the same. Silence, then, would be preferable to a cruel truth.

(c) Asteya: non-stealing and non-covetousness. These two might seem different, but according to Yoga belief, they are closely associated. Taking more than we need from mankind is a form of stealing; yearning for what others possess is a kind of stealing, and whatever we steal has the effect of shackling us and retarding our progress to self-realisation. Nothing in the universe belongs to us, but it merely loaned for the brief period of our sojourn on earth. Since the universe has limited resources, we are advised not to borrow any more than the strict necessities or we impede our spiritual progress.

(d) Aparigraha: non-acquisitiveness and the non-receiving of gifts. In the affluent society of the West, the temptations to becoming acquisitive are very great. We are pressurised on all sides by advertisements and the stigma of not keeping up with the Jones's, but the Yogi must resist and try to limit his possessions to his needs, and not his wants. It is easy to see, in this age when bribery is not only rampant, but comparatively respectable under the disguises of 'rewards', 'incentives' and 'business gifts', the dangers in accepting presents and favours from people who feel no genuine affection for us. The Yogi must refuse them. He is told that if he is to preserve his integrity and his freedom, he must not allow himself to become beholden to others. Similarly he must not make gifts except to the people he loves, and then they must be tokens of his affection and with no thought of self-advancement or of return. Receiving gifts, it is said, encourages greed and acquisitiveness and retards spiritual progress. When wishing to demonstrate his affection, the Yogi is told to give of himself, to perform personal services for his friends, but never to contemplate their being reciprocated or even appreciated.

(e) Dana: charity. As in the Biblical sense, charity is synonymous with love. It is the giving of self, the quality of consideration for, and respect of, all other beings. It must be incorporated with every thought, word and deed and it is the basis of all human relationships.

(f) Viveka: discrimination. This is another of the basic requirements of Yoga, for at every turn choices must be made between the serious and the trivial, the shadow and the substance. Often they are not so clear-cut and the Yogi is taught to learn from his own experience so that he does not repeat mistakes. Gradually he develops instinctive wisdom.

2 Niyama, the conduct towards oneself, has six observances:

(a) Soucha: cleanliness or purity. Externally it requires the body to be kept wholesome, since it is a garment to be used in the service of the mind. A proper diet must be adhered to and fasting is recommended to keep the body free from toxins. Internally the mind must not be fed on trash, frivolous chatter, puerile romances or other worthless matter which might encourage us to lapse into daydreams which, while harmless in themselves, eventually corrupt the mind by diminishing the power of thought and reason. Yoga adds that it is not what we discuss, but how we discuss it that matters. The Raja Yogi is instructed to converse with all men, and at their level, using their vocabulary. And because men of all strata are concerned with the meaning of life, they will readily respond to a discussion normally outside their range of conversation. People who have never been exposed to the ideas of philosophy might benefit and even the casual talk of everyday life might be enriched for them.

(*b*) Santosha: contentment. This does not entail indifference to the plight of others. It is a positive duty for us to do our utmost to help the less-fortunate improve their lot, and we can best do this by coming to terms with ourselves and not looking for personal gain or advancement. Contentment, too, must not be confused with complacency. It is not a self-satisfied tranquillity, but rather a deliberate counting of one's blessings, an appreciation of one's own bounty. It is not the gratification of an immediate desire, a transitory happiness which so often gives rise to another wish, another anxiety. Rather it is an absence of worry, of pain, of desire, and a equilibrium of all the senses.

(*c*) Tapas: austerity. This is a self-limiting of one's requirements, a discrimination between wants and needs. It enables one to discipline the body, recognise its appetites and restrict them, and to discipline the mind as a consequence. On the face of it, austerity seems harsh and oppressive. In fact it is a form of freedom. People who have once craved tobacco and have known genuine deprivation when none was available, have known what real freedom was once they had been cured of smoking. So it is with Yoga: conquer the appetite and freedom ensues.

(*d*) Svadhyaya: study. This can be translated by people of different religions to study their particular saviours or gods. It can be used to study the disciples or followers of Yoga, such as Ramakrishna or Buddha, or Jesus Christ who, although the founder of Christianity, embraced much of Yoga philosophy. For the non-religious or agnostic it can be adapted to study the innermost core of oneself. It is essential in this case to avoid self-recrimination when one falls short of the ideal, but to learn from past experience and from one's

observations. It is interesting to note that many modern psychologists advocate self-study as a means of avoiding and alleviating psychological disturbances.

(*e*) Ishvara-Pranidhana: devotion. This can be directed to whichever deity the Raja Yogi worships and in whatever relationship he chooses. Jesus Christ worshipped God as a father. Ramakrishna worshipped God as his mother. The wise men of the East worshipped Him as the Christ child. Arjuna in the *Gita* saw God as his friend. It does not matter. Man can relate his human feelings as he wills and if he accepts no deity, he can project his devotion towards all creation which is, in fact, the aim of Yoga.

(*f*) Brahmacharya: moderation in sex. This is often defined as continence, but is by no means the rule. It is believed that sex is the strongest and most powerful of human energies and as such it needs considerable constraint. We know that it is the force which not only preserves life but perpetuates the species. It is the instinctive sense of self-preservation of both individual men and of nations. The Raja Yogi must learn how to control it so that he can direct the power into spiritual channels. Yoga is not alone in this. The Roman Catholic Church insists on chastity and continence in its priests, and competitive sportsmen recognise that players are more likely to give of their best after a period of sexual abstention. Brahma-charya, while not insisting on total abstention, since many of its adherents will be family men, does insist that promiscuity is not only a waste of energies, but also an abuse.

3 Asanas: the postures of Hatha Yoga which must be practised by the Raja Yogi to develop the good health essential for him. Since he must be able to sit for a considerable time in one posture with relative comfort so that his physical sensations do not intrude on his mind, it is necessary for his limbs to be in good, flexible condition. The only way in which man can achieve this balance with

ease is by using the Lotus pose. If he lies down, he is liable to fall asleep. If he sits in a chair, he becomes uncomfortable with the pressure on his thighs or shoulders. Cross-legged, with his feet touching the floor he can lose his balance, so only the Lotus, with his feet resting on his thighs, affords him the stability necessary. His spine must remain erect and in a straight line from the base to the head. Only when the body is trained to be still and erect for long periods can the mind be free, and when the advanced Yogi attempts to raise the force in his spine — the Kundalini — it is essential that the body is able to sustain the Lotus pose.

4 Pranayama: breath control. As explained in Chapter 8, breath is the best means of acquiring Prana. There are three aspects:

Rechaka–exhaling
Puraka–inhaling
Kumbhaka–holding or retaining

Breath is like the fly-wheel of a machine, the machine being the body. Once the fly-wheel moves it sets the rest of the mechanism into motion. When it works perfectly, all the parts are in perfect synchronisation. To demonstrate the importance of something as apparently insignificant as the breath, there is an Asian tale.

A minister to a great king offended him and so he was imprisoned in a high tower. The devoted wife of the minister came to the foot of the tower and asked if she could help to release him. She was told to go home and secure the following: a horned beetle, some fine silk thread, some ordinary sewing thread, some stout twine and lastly some rope.

Once she had collected them she returned to the foot of the tower. Her husband called down instructions. She was to daub some honey on the beetle's horns, to fasten round its body one end of the silk thread, and to point the beetle towards the top of the tower. Naturally it crawled straight up, endeavouring to reach the honey always just ahead of it. When it had arrived at the top, she was to fasten the end of the silk to the ordinary thread.

After her husband had gently pulled this up, she had to tie the ordinary thread to the twine, and lastly the twine to the rope. And so the minister was able to free himself.

The Raja Yogi is taught by similar means to perform his daily breathing exercises. Each step, in itself, appears ineffective, but added to the whole it is strong and powerful. The Raja Yogi is advised to perform his breathing exercises in a room set aside just for that purpose, so that if he is ill or in need of extra energy he might receive it from the energies he has liberated and expended in that very room, working on the principle that, as the ripples in a pool return, so do the vibrations released by his Pranayama. When the mind and the body are stilled by Pranayama, the other limbs of Yoga can be followed. (This composure is also necessary for the practice of Kundalini Yoga when the currents are drawn upwards to the seven centres situated in the spine to afford the Yogi with occult powers beyond the range of most humans. Absolute breath control combined with erect posture and meditation are vital for this purpose.)

The Raja Yogi must spend at least half an hour each night and each morning performing Pranayama. Traditionally the measuring of time in rhythmic breathing is not done by means of numbers or heartbeats. Instead he repeats his mantra — the sacred thought or prayer usually given to him by his guru. The mantra most commonly used by people who have no guru is 'Om' — believed to be the sound which represents the cosmic force. It is repeated very slowly, the sound rising from the chest, vibrating in the larynx, the throat, against the palate and in the nasal passages so that the Yogi is enveloped in its resonance. Like many Yoga practices, the mantra is a tool to help focus his attention and it also sets up vibrations beneficial to himself and to others who come within its range.

5 Pratyahara, literally meaning 'gathering towards', is the gathering together of control of

the senses. It is a logical progression from the analysis of the senses practised by the Jnana Yogi in which he isolates each of the senses by suppressing or cutting off the others. Most of us are, to some extent, ruled by our senses: our mouths water when we smell appetising food, and often we tell ourselves it doesn't really matter if we give in to bodily demands just this once. If, however, we can overrule such physical demands so that we no longer crave undesirable substances, we can free ourselves from both the urge and the internal struggle between mind and body. Only when freed from such demands can we channel all our energies inwardly to concentrate and eventually to meditate.

The practical method of achieving such freedom from the senses is the Yogi's daily exercise of sitting in the Lotus pose, eyes half-closed, for at least half an hour, observing his own mind. He must not attempt to control or direct his thoughts, but must study and note where and how they travel. It can be compared, broadly, to the 'stream of consciousness' type of literature practised by writers such as James Joyce when the uninterrupted train of thought tumbles out without let or hindrance, drifting or leaping from apparently unrelated topics, mingling past, present and future.

It is an exercise recommended to every student of Yoga who wishes to gain insight into his own mental processes. After about a week, the mind appears to slow down. The thoughts do not flit from subject to subject but tend to penetrate more deeply each one touched. At this point each of the senses can be brought individually into operation to the exclusion of the others. All the energy can be focused so that body and mind can be concentrated on intensifying the experience of, say, the sense of smell. Once each sense can be controlled and experienced at will, it can also be 'switched off' whenever it intrudes. The one-pointedness is therefore under absolute control.

6 Dharana: concentration. Its practice is explained in greater detail in Chapter 13 which defines concentration as studying an object complete with its immediate periphery of things directly linked with it. In effect it is the daily exercise of sitting in the Lotus pose, and directing the mind first to an object, then to a concept or idea. As with all Yoga mind-control, no compulsion must be used. If the thoughts wander, they must be allowed to do so briefly, when they will of their own accord return to the object under consideration, in the belief that the denial or repudiation of any deviation would obstruct the development of thought control.

7 Dhyana: meditation and contemplation. The boundaries between the two are blurred and indistinct but, in general, meditation is reaching the core of an object, while contemplation is when the thinker and the object are merged and become a part of each other.

The Raja Yogi learns to recognise three distinct stages in each act of perception. The first, Shabda, is the ethereal vibration set up between the object and the senses of the Yogi. The second, Artha, is the motion in the nerves of the brain as it receives the meaning of what is perceived. The third, Jnana, is the knowledge and profound understanding of what is being perceived. Most of us are only aware of the combined effect but in Dhyana the Yogi is able to meditate on each stage, thus reaching the core of each act of perception.

This is considerably more complex than the so-called meditation exercises practised by most students of Yoga in the West, and it must be emphasised that it is impossible to attempt any meditation until the previous stage of concentration has been perfected. Nowadays many people speak glibly of meditating when, in fact, they mean 'thinking', and not even 'concentrating'.

8 Samadhi: absorption and self-realisation. This is a passive state when the Yogi actually becomes one with the universe. To begin with it is experienced for only short periods of time but these lengthen as the Yogi develops. He goes beyond the

concepts of good and bad and is able to reach the very centre, the very heart of everything; he and it share the same existence and both are mere parts of the universe, just as a person's limbs and organs are a part of him. The Yogi absorbs the object being studied but he neither influences it nor colours it with his own self. Thus it is sometimes referred to as 'absorption'.

Those who achieve Samadhi see God, or the cosmic force, clearly in everything. When Ramakrishna was questioned about his own experiences he explained that he could see God more clearly than he could see his own disciples, and he meant it literally. This is the union of Yoga, the true knowledge which the Yogi sees and from which comes absolute peace.

The first five limbs of Raja Yoga, are in preparation for the latter three which can be grouped together and termed Sanyama, for they comprise a combined action of concentrating on an object (concentration), observing the core of it and becoming at one with it (meditation and contemplation) and having the ability to be at one with all creation (absorption).

When this final stage is reached, and the Yogi has arrived at the hub of the wheel, his true spiritual life can begin. It is believed that he develops psychic faculties which enable him to penetrate time and space and to emit a radiance which can help and guide people over great distances. The traditional Yoga acceptance of reincarnation concludes that once Samadhi is reached, the Yogi is free from having to live out further lives on earth.

Patience and perseverance not just in this life, but in every life, is essential and is illustrated in the story of Narada, the Yogi who was mentioned in Chapter 3. He was on his way walking towards heaven when he met a Yogi sitting in the woods meditating. The Yogi had sat for so long and in such deep thought that a colony of white ants had built their mound around him. When he found that Narada was on his way to heaven, the disconsolate

Yogi asked if he would find out from God how long it would be before he could be freed from his trials and achieve Samadhi. Narada went on his way and eventually came upon a volatile man who veered between extremes of elation and despondency. He too asked Narada to question God about when he would achieve freedom.

After having reached heaven and now on his way home, Narada called on the Yogi in the ant hill and told him that God had said he had four more earthly lives to live before he would be free. The man groaned and shook his head, dreading his future. When Narada arrived at the other man, who was still leaping from one experience to another, he told him he had as many lives to live as there were leaves on yonder tree. The tree was in full foliage but the man jumped for joy. He was delighted that eventually, no matter how far off, he would attain freedom and he thanked Narada warmly. At that moment a voice spoke out from heaven informing the man that he was to be freed that very moment. His perseverance and lack of self-discouragement had done more for him than all the stoicism of the Yogi.

Samadhi is the ultimate goal of the Yogi. Buddhists refer to it as Nirvana and mystics throughout the ages have told how they could transcend time and space. Most major religions recognise such a state although they give different accounts of it.

Part Two

THE PRACTICE OF HATHA YOGA

7 Relaxation

It is believed that more illness and disease is caused by stress than by any other single cause, and taken to its logical conclusion, stress is the result of the inability to relax, to 'let go'. Animals, in their natural state, avoid it by taking action when presented with problems. A cornered rat will fight, a threatened bird will fly away, and the weaker of two contesting wolves will be allowed to make its escape.

Unfortunately civilisation imposes restrictions on our innate instincts. The man who is unhappy at his work might be forced by economic reasons to put up with his state, just as the housewife who must stay at home looking after toddlers when she would prefer to go out to work, has to postpone her ambitions and accept her frustration.

But if we can recapture the animal method of relaxation during certain periods of each day, severe anxiety and stress are prevented from building up into unmanageable proportions. When this build-up is allowed to happen, the body mechanism is liable to rebel. It releases excessive amounts of harmful secretions, some of which can induce heart damage and activate the numerous bacteria and viruses co-existing within us but not causing illness so long as the body is not subjected to over-strain, and so instigate such complaints as rheumatism, cancer and stomach ulcers, as well as psychiatric disturbances.

All animals are prone to stress diseases which, in their natural habitat, could be instinctively avoided, but which can prove killers in captivity. Wallabies, for example, if roughly handled in zoos, will develop a fatal illness known as 'lumpy jaw' from which they die within a few days.

The Chinese say we all carry within us the seeds of our own destruction and nowhere is this more true than in the stress diseases so prevalent today. The Yoga way of relaxation is remarkably simple to learn and once acquired it can be practised by anyone whatever their age or their state of health. Its benefits are instantaneous.

There is a Greek-Cypriot proverb that says 'Work is hard, no work is harder' and this is true of Yoga relaxation. It may seem contradictory, but it is more difficult to keep still than to move. Observe just how much the average person fidgets and changes his position while he is supposed to be at ease. It is not easy to locate the seat of the tension. In some people it is in their hands which seem to tighten and clench themselves involuntarily. In others it is at the base of the skull in the nape of the neck, while in others it is in their jaw — they grind their teeth. In order to find the exact spot within ourselves (not easy if for many years such places have been constantly tense so that we have forgotten what it is like to be at ease) we must temporarily increase the tension before relaxation can be achieved. Working, or even resting, when tense is like trying to ride a bicycle with the brakes on. One force is pushing against the other and any action becomes more difficult and increases the residual tension.

The first step is to lie down on a mat or rug on a hard floor. As with all Yoga exercises, any clothing worn must be loose and light with no constrictions at waist, neck or wrists. If possible the exercises should be performed out of doors or else in a well-ventilated room. Before starting the actual exercises, most Westerners will need to flatten their spines, for most of us find that when lying flat on our backs the spine does not touch the floor along its whole length. We can slide a hand in the hollow behind the waist. Easterners, especially workers who are used to carrying weights on their heads, don't usually have this problem and Yoga exercises and poses can best be performed when this hollow is minimised.

The way to do it is:

1 Lie flat on the floor, face upwards.

2 Bend the knees and bring them up to the chest.

3 Clasp the knees with both arms, close to the chest, for a few moments.

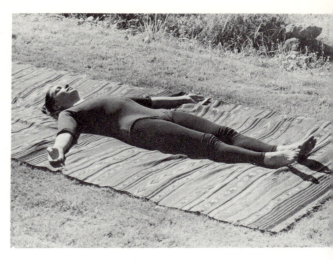

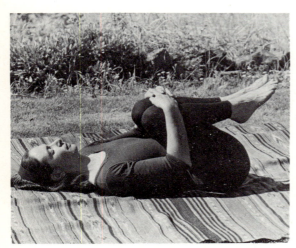

Spine-flattening exercise

4 Slowly lower the legs to the floor and at the same time try to press the spine against the floor. It sometimes helps to press the palm of one hand against the navel during (4) and to open the mouth and exhale sharply, making 'ha-ha' sounds while pressing the spine against the floor. This exercise should be repeated three times.

Now, still lying flat on the back, slowly breathe in and at the same time raise the outstretched arms from the sides of the body to as far as they will reach above the head, remembering to slide them so that they never lose contact with the floor. Holding the breath, stretch the arms upwards and

the legs — toes pointed — downwards so that the entire body is taut. Give a long, slow pull, then slowly lower the arms to the side while exhaling, and making sure that they slide along the floor. Repeat this three times.

The first classic Yoga pose, or asana, to be done is the Savasana or Dead pose which puts the whole nervous system at rest and slows down the pulse and breathing. One hour of this exercise is believed to do the body more good than an average night's sleep. It must be performed at the beginning and again at the end of each day's Yoga exercise session, and should be interspersed with the exercises.

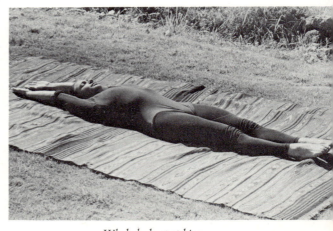

Whole body stretching

SAVASANA: DEAD POSE

1 Lie flat on the back, arms against the sides, eyes closed.

2 Wriggle the toes, moving them as if they were trying to pick up a pencil and at the same time put your consciousness into them, thinking only of them. This is the first lesson in concentration.

3 Relax the toes, still thinking of them. Pause for a few seconds.

4 Slightly raise the ankles from the floor and rotate them for about five seconds, again keeping the mind on them.

5 Relax the ankles, still thinking of them. Pause for a few seconds.

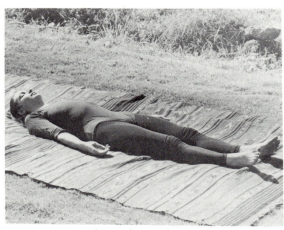

The Dead pose: Savasana

Move upwards this way, tensing and relaxing the calves, then the knees, the hips, abdomen, the fingers (with a clawing motion), the fists (which should be clenched several times), the wrists (rotating them), the elbows, the shoulders, the chest, the neck (which should be lifted slightly and rotated) and finally the face (stretching into grimaces), opening and tensing eyes by rolling them, twitching the nose, ears, scalp and eyebrows, and opening the jaws as if in a yawn. As each part is exercised, the mind should dwell on that part as in (2) above.

Not only are the limbs, muscles and joints relaxed, but the internal organs are flushed out. If you press forefinger and thumb together, the blood is extruded from the tips. Once the pressure is removed, an increased flow of blood rushes to the deprived parts, and so it is with internal organs many of which have insufficient supply of blood because of faulty posture or inadequate exercise. Once we get used to the sensation of being without tension, it is easier for us to recognise it when and where it arises, so that wherever we are if we find our muscles stiffening, we can consciously stiffen them even more and then relax and so avoid starting the cycle of tension again.

When every part of the body has been tensed and then allowed to relax, lie perfectly still on the floor, eyes closed, and mentally go over every muscle, joint and limb to see if any feel at all tense or slightly unrelaxed. If so, tense the parts individually as in (2) and (3) above. Now lie still for a minimum of ten minutes. Imagine you are lying on a very soft bed — much easier than it sounds, for although the floor will feel hard and unyielding for the first week or so, the body soon adapts itself. After a month or so it is quite usual to experience a sense of weightlessness, as if floating or sinking, and students unprepared for this are sometimes a little afraid, the sensations being unknown to them. This is real relaxation and even greater benefit is achieved if the position can be maintained for half an hour. If during the relaxation period tension arises in any part of the body, tense it and then relax it. But do not deliberately look for tension, rather let the mind think of other things.

Experienced Yogis can deliberately massage and stimulate their internal organs by means of putting their consciousness into the parts, and all of us benefit from the greater control we develop through the practice of relaxation. Nervous tension can be as bad as physical, and Yogis are advised to study themselves to determine the cause. Perhaps a woman feels socially inferior and finds herself blushing in company. Yoga teaches her to evaluate herself so that she can regard herself dispassionately. She must learn to stop comparing herself to others; she must accept herself for what she is. By all means she should try to improve herself if she wishes, but she must not devalue herself. This is contrary to what most of us have been conditioned to do. As little children we are compared — often to our discredit — with others by teachers and parents. Many schools work on the competitive spirit, hence the 'house' system, examinations and sports contests.

Yoga is against all these methods. Each man must find himself and having done so, should accept what he is. Naturally he is urged to achieve his potential, but only with regard to himself and not with the aim of beating other people. Fear of failure is at the root of much nervous tension and since the Yogi learns to accept either failure or success with equanimity, such fear is unknown.

Possibly many middle-aged people are happier for having come to terms with themselves without ever having studied Yoga. They accept that they will never be a great artist or a concert pianist, and they stop berating or driving themselves, knowing that they have insufficient talent. Those, however, who refuse to face up to their own limitations are the people most likely to suffer from stress complaints, and it is possibly they who are in greater need of Yoga.

8 Prana

As with all Yoga teaching, there are no absolute rules laid down for the acquisition of Prana, only guidelines for the student to accept or modify depending on how far he wishes to adapt himself or his lifestyle. One thing is certain, however, whether you devote your life to Yoga principles or are completely ignorant of them, you will inevitably imbibe a certain amount of Prana because it is believed that life cannot be sustained without it. What Yoga does insist on, however, is that you will enjoy a healthier and fuller life if you consciously add to your daily intake and learn how to store it as vitality or stamina.

The main sources of Prana are:

1 air
2 sunshine
3 sleep
4 water
5 food

It follows that the purer the air, food or water, the more Prana it will contain and the healthier your body, the more it can store against times of great activity, mental or physical, and against times of unavoidable stress.

Although no machine or instrument has been invented that can detect the presence of Prana, those who have practised Yoga claim they are aware of it. So it is with certain odours which even now can be detected by the human nose in minute proportions which so far no scientific apparatus can register. People who have learnt to increase their intake of Prana are invariably aware of the added sense of well-being and of the reserves of strength unknown to them before. Born healers such as magnetic or faith healers are supposed to be possessors of superior amounts, and the ingestion of Prana is at the root of all mental and physical health.

AIR

Correct breathing, using the whole of the lungs, is the most important single means of taking in Prana (see Chapter 10), but pollution in most of the world's cities where large sections of the population live, is an ever-increasing hazard. Wherever possible, city-dwellers should go into the country, by the seaside or, best of all, into the mountains where generally air is of far better quality. Unfortunately there is insufficient understanding of what constitutes fresh air. Every summer weekend country roads, often jammed with traffic, are lined with picnickers who leave the polluted air of the city to breathe in the even more polluted air only yards away from heavy traffic.

Instead of sitting in a lay-by they should leave the main road and if there is no access to a field, stay in a quiet lane or go for a walk. There is usually more Prana and oxygen in the air near forests for trees purify surrounding air, a fact well-known to those who built sanatoria in the woods.

SUNSHINE

The sun is the greatest source of vitality and energy without which no life could exist on this planet. Early morning sunshine is preferable to that of midday and, incidentally, produces a deeper tan with less burning. This theory of early sun being more beneficial applies to plants as well as to humans. It has been noticed that strawberries under cloches running from north to south ripen days — even weeks — earlier on the east-facing side than on the west. Traditionally Yogis the world over are advised to do their daily exercises in the morning facing east, out of doors if possible. In many Indian schools the children start the day performing Suryanamaskar — salutation to the sun. It is a physical prayer to the sun and incorporates several Yoga poses performed in unbroken succession.

There is an element of symbolism in early morning activity. A new day is beginning, a new start. The body is refreshed after sleep, the air clean and refreshed with dew, and while the exercises can be performed at any hour, students are advised to try doing them as early as possible in the morning. Contrary to popular belief, sunbathing is not recommended except when done early or late in the day, in shade or in dappled sunshine. Otherwise it is considered to be both exhausting and ageing.

SLEEP

The third source of Prana is sleep which, according to Yoga, is more beneficial if taken before midnight. This echoes the old wives' tales of one hour's sleep before midnight being worth two afterwards. The modern science of biorhythmics shows that some medicines will have twice the effect if taken at a particular hour. More people die at 4am than at any other time. Perhaps the body can gain more benefit from sleep, therefore, when it is taken before midnight.

It is a fact that primitive peoples obey their instincts and begin their sleep as soon as darkness falls. To find out if we gain by going to bed earlier and getting up earlier, students are advised to give it a trial for two or three weeks. Go to bed at the normal time but set an alarm clock for 6am. For the first few days it is likely that the body will

suffer fatigue. Since we go to bed late and get up earlier than usual, we might be constantly tired, but after a few days it becomes easier to go to bed early and so to form a new habit. Those who have tried it claim that their memory improves and that study done in the early morning is more easily retained. If social activities or work make this experiment impossible, the new sleep pattern can be tried during holidays. In any event it is worthwhile trying to get to bed before midnight, even if only by an hour.

To get the most benefit from sleep, we are advised not to eat or drink for at least two hours before going to bed, a practice widely followed in other countries such as France. Hard mattresses and no pillow — or at most, one thin one — help to keep the spine flat and straight so that the organs can fulfil their work unhindered and undistorted. If possible the head of the bed should point towards the north and the foot south. This puts the sleeper in harmony with the flow of currents and magnetic forces from the earth. Some Yogis claim they can feel the difference once they are attuned to receiving these currents.

The amount of sleep required should be discovered by self-experimentation, and while a lack of sleep will produce disorientation, hallucinations and profound physical distress, too much sleep can stunt both mental and physical activity. Only by individual trials can the correct amount be determined.

WATER

It is becoming increasingly difficult to gain access to clean, unadulterated drinking water, especially in towns and cities. Chlorine and other chemicals must be added to protect the population from typhoid and cholera, and recently there has been considerable controversy because of the addition of mass-medication with fluoride. Because the quantity of water drunk varies widely from person to person, those who stand to gain from fluoride, that is, young children, might be getting insufficient while those on whom it is wasted, the rest of the population, might be getting too much. The question remains largely academic since few of us have any choice in the matter. Nevertheless we should resist the practice of mass-medication by means of water supplies, especially where more selective methods, such as adding fluoride to children's milk or by giving them tablets, would be both cheaper and more efficient.

Another problem of civilisation is the incidence of old, lead water-pipes. People living in property with such plumbing are advised to run the tap for at least five minutes to flush away the excess lead deposits before drinking or boiling the water. In all cases we are advised to drink clean, spring water whenever we visit mountains.

Few of us drink enough plain water; we drink it in tea, coffee or soft drinks, but it is a simple way of cleaning the system and in fasting (see Chapter 9) it is essential to drink large quantities to flush out impurities. Water provides amounts of Prana in other ways. There are considerable quantities in the air near waterfalls, lakes and the seaside.

Scientists in many countries have shown that negatively ionised air brings relief in respiratory complaints such as asthma and bronchitis. It inhibits the spread of infection and gives people a sense of well-being. Ions are continuously created in nature by ultra-violet light and by the splitting of water droplets as in waterfalls or sea waves, and while there are machines to simulate these conditions, they are there for everyone to enjoy in such regions. Thus the continental habit of taking a cure at spas may be a very sound practice.

A lesser source of Prana, but not to be dismissed, is by a period of voluntary silence. It is no use staying at home and vowing not to speak for a day; the resultant tensions and frustrations would do more harm than good. Better to go out into the country, perhaps for a long walk alone, where there is no temptation to speak. The religious retreats visited by many people in search of peace is yet another example of people practising Yoga without even being aware of it.

FOOD

The dedicated Yogi is a vegetarian — he drinks no alcohol, takes no drugs or stimulants and does not smoke. For most people this is too rigorous a regime and because there is no dogma, students are asked to regard the recommendations simply as guidelines to be aimed at and worked towards.

We must understand that we are what we eat. Try feeding a racehorse on unsuitable food and it will not be able to give of its best. This fact is well-known by zoologists, especially when animals are removed from their natural habitat where their instincts would guide them to the correct food. Once they are in zoos and must depend on man, their health and performance varies in direct proportion to the type of food they are given. So it is with humans. Most of us have lost the instincts which could direct us to the right food in the right quantity, thus nearly half of all adults in the developed countries are overweight.

Yoga students are advised to get to know their own appetites. Pause before nibbling between meals or accepting an extra portion at dinner, and see if you are prompted by hunger or by the wish to savour the taste. If in doubt, drink water between meals or find something to do to take the mind off the appetite. In a short time the stomach can be retrained and it will actually shrink so that it feels full sooner. In this way healthy eating habits are formed.

The principal guidelines for Yoga students are:
(a) All food should be as naturally produced as possible.
(b) Food should be as little tampered with as possible.
(c) There should be a minimum of stimulants in the diet.
(d) Vegetarianism should be developed.

(a) It is becoming increasingly difficult to find food which has been grown without the use of chemical fertilisers and insecticides, despite the damage which is done to the body by these additives. The liver, which acts as a filter, is often the first part of the body to be injured, making it less efficient in containing the toxins. But because of the resulting ill-health and possible degeneration of the cells, it is worthwhile to go to some trouble to find naturally produced foods.

Some cities now have whole-food shops where the products are guaranteed organically grown, but those people who have no such access are urged, if they possibly can, to grow their own. Even the smallest garden can produce effective amounts of fruit and vegetables, and if there is no area available for the exclusive use of a kitchen garden, many vegetables have beautiful flowers and foliage and could well be grown among orthodox decorative plants. Red cabbage, purple sprouting broccoli with its pretty yellow flowers, purple beans and even the humble carrot could enhance any herbaceous border. A small compost heap would supply all the necessary fertiliser for little or no cost, and insecticides are unnecessary. When plants are healthy they are usually free from, or can withstand, attacks from pests, and if pests were indeed evident, non-poisonous sprays like derris and pyrethrum could be used.

Having tasted organically grown produce eaten straight from the garden, it is unlikely that anyone would again be satisfied with sprayed commercial products; and because the vitamin C content — and Prana — starts diminishing from the moment the fruit and vegetables are cut or plucked, it is vital to eat them as fresh as possible. Years ago many countrywomen used to take a pot of boiling water with them when they went into the garden to gather their peas and beans. Without going so far, it is advisable to gather food at the last possible moment. In addition it should be cooked by steaming it in a pan with a tight lid rather than by boiling with water, and, of course, for the shortest possible time. Those vegetables which can be eaten raw, such as carrots, tomatoes, celery and cabbage provide greater amounts of both vitamins and Prana, and some raw vegetable or fruit should be taken at each meal.

Fresh dairy food is as necessary as fresh vegetables and where there is any choice, that which is preserved in any way such as sterilised milk should be accepted only as a last resort. Cream cheese, therefore, is better than hard cheese, and free-range eggs are always preferable to battery eggs. The latter, if eaten at all, should be taken sparingly. Factory-farmed poultry has to be fed large amounts of antibiotics because hens raised in such unnatural conditions would succumb to disease and stress if they were not kept tranquillised constantly. In addition they are given hormones and growth stimulants which tend to remain in the eggs and and in the poultry flesh. In order of preference the best food is fresh, followed by frozen and lastly, preserved and canned.

(b) As well as avoiding too much cooking which destroys the goodness, we should beware of food which has been tampered with before it reaches us. The most obvious examples are bread and rice, both of which are largely de-natured to make them look white. The wheat germ is removed and replaced with chalk in all except 100 per cent wholemeal flour. Other additives are put into the refined flour to restore some of the vitamins, but most of them are chemicals. It seems absurd to remove natural properties and wheatgerm to replace them with dubious inferior products, but this is the law of the land. It is interesting to note that during the last war when the national loaf was less white and therefore contained more of the whole wheat, the nation's health (and teeth) improved, despite the strain of air raids and the shortages of many foods. If possible Yoga students should eat wholemeal bread, making their own if they can — it is surprisingly easy, far easier, for example, than baking cakes. Brown unpolished rice should be preferred to white.

There are 1,500 chemical additives in general use today which are either added to food or which form artificial substitutes, and even substitutes for substitutes, including thirty permitted dyes. Although these are within the law of this country, some other countries ban their use as being known to produce cancer and are suspected of causing such degenerative diseases as arteriosclerosis, cataracts, arthritis and heart disease. It follows, therefore, that we should never buy a can or a packet of food without first reading the label. If there is any choice, take the food with the fewest number of chemical additives.

(c) As well as obvious drugs — alcohol, tea and coffee — one of the main stimulants used today is sugar. A food of civilisation, it has already made inroads into the teeth of developed nations and is now suspected of being connected with the high incidence of coronary complaints common to people who eat large amounts. Ideally children should not be given sugar or sweets. Those in underdeveloped countries who do not taste chocolate until puberty usually do not acquire the addiction to it.

The rest of us should endeavour to retrain our tastebuds. As with all Yoga teaching, the change should be gradual. Begin by taking half portions of sugar in tea and coffee, lessening the allowance over a period of weeks until we take none. It may take six weeks or longer before hitherto sweet drinks are platable without sugar, but after that it is usual to find sweetened drinks unpalatable. As well as the sugar in tea and coffee, there is considerable 'hidden' in foods such as puddings, desserts, biscuits and cakes. These too, should be decreased and if sugar is used at all, brown is preferable to white. It is a fallacy that sugar provides energy. Sustained energy is provided by the consumption of vegetables and fresh or dried fruit, or by eating wild honey. Normal commercial honey is likely to be produced by bees fed on sugar and is therefore similar to eating the sugar itself.

Other stimulants like alcohol, tea and coffee should be taken as little as possible, and the amounts can be decreased by dilution, making tea and coffee weaker. It is advisable, too, to try alternative drinks, such as fruit or vegetable juices and vegetable extracts available at health-food shops for hot drinks.

(d) Yogis are, ideally, vegetarians because the first principle of Yama — conduct towards others — is non-violence. The reverence for life precludes the taking of it and by foregoing meat, the Yogi eliminates one source of killing. The second reason is that they believe it is less healthy to eat meat, particularly nowadays when its production is so dubious. It is quite usual for stall-fed cattle to be given hormones and aureomycin during the period of growth, tranquillisers to calm them on their way to the slaughter-house, and an injection of antibiotics immediately before death to help the meat keep in cold storage and become more tender. Many of these residues are eaten in the subsequent meat.

Yoga teaches that we do not need enormous amounts of protein unless we are growing, and that we can get more than enough from cheese, eggs, nuts and pulses such as peas and lentils. It is better that a meat-eater should not become a vegetarian suddenly. He is advised to begin by lessening the amount of meat eaten by starting with one or two meatless days a week. Presently he stops eating meat but continues to eat fish and poultry. Eventually he becomes a true vegetarian, the whole transition having taken two or more years. To change a diet suddenly might shock the system and perhaps cause psychological disturbances. Although some people can abstain from meat-eating at once with no ill effects, it is not advisable for most to do so suddenly.

Variety and balance is as important as quality and only by eating a wide assortment of fruit and vegetables can one be certain of acquiring all the minerals and vitamins necessary for good health. Too much of any one food is discouraged, and students are advised to experiment for themselves but to avoid developing fads. Rigid diets should be avoided and since each person is unique, each must decide what to eat and in what proportions.

To those who experience digestive disturbances, the four counsels are:

1 Chew each mouthful of food well and slowly, since much of the digestion should begin with the saliva in the mouth. This practice of chewing slowly is a help in reducing the appetite.

2 Never eat when tired, angry or distressed. This is sound physiological advice instinctively followed by animals whose very lives might depend on their being able to flee or to fight. When the organism is in the process of digesting food, other activities are slowed down or inhibited.

3 No drink should be taken with or immediately after meals because they tend to dilute the digestive juices. If necessary, drinks can be taken an hour before a meal, or in-between meals.

4 Never eat at the same meal-time starch food with protein, that is, do not eat potatoes with cheese, or egg and toast. Nor should you eat acid or citrus fruit with starch. So if you have potatoes with one course, don't have pineapple for dessert. It is believed that these combinations war with each other as each requires a different digestive enzyme which cannot operate efficiently at the same time.

Within a week of practising these combinations, the digestion should improve. The above are counsels of perfection and students of Yoga are expected to make their own decisions as to which they accept.

One counsel which can be followed by most people is to rest for a while and not undertake hard physical or mental work immediately after meals. The body has to concentrate its energies on assimilating the food and if other demands are made on it, the stomach is deprived of blood and muscle-tone, resulting in digestive disturbance or worse.

One of the earliest experiments which proved this was performed by a wealthy Roman who had two of his slaves lavishly fed. He made one work very hard immediately after the meal, while the other had to rest in bed. An hour or so later he had them both killed so that the contents of their stomachs could be examined. The one who had worked during his last hour had barely begun to digest his food, while the stomach of the other showed that the food was partially digested. Many Latins take a siesta after their main meal of the day, and while this is not strictly necessary, it is advisable to avoid vigorous exercise for an hour after eating.

9 Fasting

Although Prana is not absorbed by the body during a fast, the organism is revitalised and brought to such a state of health that subsequently it can increase its intake. Throughout history man has fasted, either for health or for religion. It is mentioned by Homer and in the Bible, and without doubt primitive man practised it. In the animal world it is of supreme importance. Even domestic cats and dogs will refuse to eat and will drink only water when they are unwell, yet most of us seem to think we should die if we failed to have three regular meals a day. Most of the advanced zoos in the world refrain from feeding many of the animals for one day each week, fasting them, in fact, to keep them in the peak of condition.

In itself it is not a cure, but when one realises the continuous work having to be performed by the digestive organs both by day and by night in those who eat just before going to bed, it is reasonable to expect that an occasional respite would benefit the whole body and give its resources a chance to repair and heal themselves. Energy that is expended on digestive processes can be diverted to the actions of elimination, and when no food is eaten, the body soon draws upon its stored reserves. When this fat in the tissues is liquidated, toxins which may have been stored up along with it, sometimes for years, are also released.

It follows that anyone feeling off-colour or perhaps starting a cold, would find immediate relief if they were to refuse all food and all drinks except water. Similarly, overweight people could expect a weight loss of up to six pounds a day for the first few days of fasting, weight which would not be immediately regained if they kept to a moderately low-calorie diet afterwards.

Naturally some self-discipline is required, but usually only for the first day or two, after which appetite disappears as the body begins to draw on its reserves. This is a faculty developed by nature to enable animals to withstand periods of famine without resorting to eating unsuitable foods. Although many of our primitive instincts have disappeared, the one to withstand shortage of food for a time is still present, although it has been overlaid by our habit of eating by the clock almost from the moment of birth.

So efficient is the body mechanism, even in sick people, that in a supervised fast lasting as long as sixty days, no sign of vitamin deficiency such as beriberi, scurvy or rickets arise, demonstrating that the body reserves are perfectly balanced to provide the right amount of necessary requirements when food is withdrawn. However, it is inadvisable for anyone to fast for longer than three complete days without supervision, if only because most of us cannot recognise within ourselves the exact moment when the body has used up its reserves. Animals and some people feel a return of hunger at this point, and if this were to be ignored, as it might in an inexperienced person fasting alone, harm could be done when the body begins to consume itself. This is where fasting ends and starvation begins.

In many health clinics sick patients as well as healthy frequently fast for upwards of three weeks until their systems are completely cleared of accumulated toxins, toxins which may have caused such varied complaints as asthma, rheumatism, high blood-pressure and stomach ulcers. But they are under constant medical supervision and, moreover, spend most of the time resting in bed.

Fasting is perfectly safe for everyone, so long as certain rules are followed — the first is, we repeat, to limit the period to three days at the most.

The second is to take only water, preferably either lukewarm or at room temperature. Both iced or boiling water must be avoided as they cause a shock to the digestive organs. Any quantity of cool water can be drunk at any time of the night or day.

The third rule is to prepare yourself mentally and physically for the fast. Any fear or trepidation will make it more difficult and as boredom often manifests itself as a feeling of hunger, some interesting pastime or occupation should be provided. It is a help if two friends can stay together and fast at the same time for mutual encouragement and support — as in group therapy — neither wanting to give in first. Obviously it would be foolish to spend much time cooking for other people, reading about food or being within the range of kitchen odours.

The fourth rule is to rest. For a short fast of twenty-four hours, light work can be done, but no long walks or heavy work. For a three-day fast it is best to stay close to the house, to rest, but not necessarily stay in bed, for several periods during the day and to undertake nothing that requires intense concentration, at least during the first fasts. Later when you have experienced two or three fasts, you may find that studying not only becomes easier, but welcome, since the brain and memory improve considerably in performance once the body is rid of its toxins. Those who are elderly or ill should spend most of the time in bed.

The fifth rule is to keep warm, for those on a fast tend to feel the cold more. Extra clothes on the bed, perhaps a hot water-bottle, and warm socks during the day are necessary.

The sixth is bathing. To prevent the pores being clogged with the toxins which are being eliminated all over the body, warm baths should be taken for a few minutes daily, or a complete sponge-down would do.

The seventh rule is not so much a rule as a piece of advice. In spring or summer it helps to sunbathe for ten minutes either early or late in the day. Since the body is ingesting very little Prana, it is vitalising to gather some from the sun, but not if the weather is too hot or too cold.

Lastly some Yogis advocate the administration of an enema. This is a controversial issue. While some swear by it, many do not, an argument repeated among orthodox physicians. Certainly an enema helps to remove toxins quickly, but it is often better not to assist elimination in such an artifical way as it removes necessary mucous from the intestines. It can be left to the individual and is not of vital importance.

To introduce yourself to fasting for the first time, it is as well to begin slowly. Those who always eat breakfast might try replacing it with just fresh fruit once a week. Then, one day a week, they could try having both lunch and breakfast of only fruit and a few weeks later try a whole day on just fruit. It is important to remember that although the quantity of fruit taken is unlimited, it must be eaten only at the three regular intervals and not nibbled at any time. Water can be drunk in between, but nothing else, neither tea, coffee, medicine nor alcohol. A variation could be to organise the days as above, but take fresh fruit juices instead of solid fruit. But do not delude yourself that this is fasting; it is not. A fast means taking *nothing* but water.

The first fast might begin after the evening meal at six o'clock. Take nothing except water that evening. The next morning and all day have nothing but water in unlimited amounts until six o'clock at night. Then have about a half pint of fresh fruit juice as a substitute for the evening meal. The next morning the breakfast must consist only of fresh fruit, the lunch of raw vegetables or salad and the evening meal can be normal.

The gentle breaking of a fast is of utmost importance, since damage can be done to the system if solid food is taken too suddenly. The body must have time to change gear, so to speak, and start up its digestive processes slowly. When a three-day fast is taken the same routine must be followed but for a longer, more gradual period. Thus:

three days on nothing but water

the fourth day, nothing but fresh fruit juices *only at meal times*

the fifth day, nothing but fresh fruit *only at meal times*

the sixth day nothing but raw grated vegetables and salads *only at meal times*

the seventh day a normal mixed diet

Throughout the whole seven-day period, water can be drunk freely, but it is apparent that although the fast itself lasts only for the first three days, the process of eliminating its stored-up toxins is actually proceeding the whole week. No matter how well you feel after the three-day fast and no matter how hungry you feel — and hunger returns as soon as the first drink of fruit juice breaks the fast — the above regime *must* be strictly observed. Even when people have been on the verge of death after prolonged starvation, a far cry from the results of even the longest fast, they cannot be given much food suddenly or they would certainly die.

In the last war the released prisoners of German concentration camps had to be fed minute portions of light food for some months although they actually wept and begged for more, and sailors who have been shipwrecked have had to undergo similar rehabilitation before their stomach and digestive organs could cope with normal portions.

A general rule of thumb is that the period of the actual fast should be equalled by the gradual return to normality. Any speeding-up would be harmful and would more than nullify the benefit obtained from the fast. Clearly such a change in the eating pattern will produce symptoms, some of them unpleasant, but none of them harmful or dangerous once they are recognised. Some experience a general feeling of weakness on the second or third day, but this is by no means universal and it seldom lasts more than twenty-four hours. In some there is a bout of nausea or vomiting which is to be welcomed and even encouraged as it hastens the elimination and you feel much better immediately after the attack has passed. People who have kept dogs or cats will recognise these symptoms, for many animals actually eat inedible grasses to make themselves vomit.

Headaches, bad breath, a coated tongue and a foul taste in the mouth are other manifestations of the toxins being liberated from the tissues, and they can be made more acceptable by copious drinks of water. Weight loss has already been mentioned, but it is interesting to note that people who want to gain weight can actually do so after fasting. This is because their digestive tract has been in an unhealthy condition and has been allowing food to pass through the body without divesting itself of the essential nourishment. Once the digestive system is healthy, it can extract the benefits from the food and there is then no need to eat such large quantities of food as before.

Some sleeplessness seems inevitable, if only because little exercise is being taken, but you are advised not to lie awake worrying about it — probably you will feel wide-awake anyhow. Better to sit up and read and if necessary take a nap during the daytime. People who have been in the habit of taking sleeping pills can often completely master the habit during a fast, finding that they can sleep naturally afterwards.

Diarrhoea, constipation and catarrh are other ways by which the body removes its stored-up waste and is no cause for alarm. It seems a little odd that when the body is taking in no food more seems to be excreted, but it is explained by the fact that without having to expend energy on digesting, the organism can concentrate on elimination. For the first day or two the urine is often dark and concentrated, but this gradually lightens as the body is cleansed.

Not all the symptoms are unpleasant and, indeed, many people experience only the nicer ones. There is a tremendous feeling of well-being so that you might want to attempt some vigorous exercise. This must, of course, be resisted for the heart might be damaged if, in a long fast, physical energy was used. Gentle exercise and the less-strenuous Yoga asanas are beneficial in the one- to three-day fasts recommended here, but no spring-cleaning, gardening or sports!

People who normally overeat and/or feel sluggish after meals find themselves more able to concentrate and study during a fast. The memory invariably improves, hearing and eyesight sharpen, particularly in those who fast regularly and so do not accumulate much toxin, and those who habitually suffer from indigestion or rheumatic pains can find great relief without having to take drugs — a matter of some importance now that more than £15 million is spent in Britain each year on digestive aids.

Unless one can afford to have a prolonged fast at a health centre or otherwise under expert supervision, it is advisable to make a habit of fasting regularly. Some fast one day every week, perhaps at weekends when they can stay at home. Others have a three-day fast one weekend every two or three months. The first one is the hardest, if only because it is something strange, but it is worth the attempt for the great improvement in general health and increased resistance against illness. Of course, the progress cannot be expected to be maintained for long unless a reasonable diet is made a permanent feature of life.

10   Pranayama
or Breathing Exercises

Of all the practices of Hatha Yoga, none is more important than correct breathing and in fact people who for some reason or other are not able to perform the postures, derive considerable benefit just from the breathing exercises or Pranayama.

In his natural state man, like animals, needs no instruction. If he did not take in sufficient oxygen he would not have the stamina and health to outrace danger. Without the warm clothes and heated shelters of civilisation he would not be able to survive the occasional extremes of even a temperate climate, so the vast variety of exercise he would have to take just to stay alive would ensure good co-ordination and efficient circulation.

The price of civilisation is that we have lost these abilities or else we have allowed them to fall into disuse. It is seldom necessary for us to exert ourselves physically unless we follow some sport. Design of clothes is such that many of us have constrictions at waist or neck, and our way of life means that much of our time is spent leaning over machines, desks or driving-wheels. All this affects the efficiency of the lungs, hence they are often functioning at only one-fifth of their total capacity. To appreciate the effect this has on our entire system, it is necessary to understand a little of the mechanism and what the air we breathe does for us.

Blood starts out from the arteries of the heart bright red and full of properties essential to health. It returns by way of the veins, sluggish, bluish and laden with the impurities it has gathered from the body during its journey. Its final lap is through the lungs where it is distributed to air cells. As soon as a breath is taken, the oxygen comes into contact with the blood through the thin walls of the lungs' hair-like blood vessels. A form of combustion takes place when the blood takes in the oxygen and in turn releases gas generated from the impurities which the blood has collected as it travelled round the body.

Once it is purified and red again, the blood returns to the heart before setting off once more on its life-saving mission. In twenty-four hours something like 35,000 pints of blood pass through each pair of lungs and are cleansed and re-energised by the breaths we take. It follows that unless we inhale sufficient oxygen, there is considerable danger that the blood is not efficiently purified and that it must return to the heart and travel round the body carrying waste products. Since digestion depends, to a certain extent, on supplies of fresh oxygen meeting food and causing yet another form of combustion, it can be readily appreciated how many stomach troubles can be directly attributed to poor breathing.

Not only is the quantity of air breathed important, but so is the quality. People who breathe through their mouths are by-passing the best filter system of all, the nose. It is equipped with tiny hairs to trap impurities, as anyone can see who blows his nose after an hour in a city or in a room with an open fire. It is capable of warming the air to the exact temperature preferred by the lungs and of humidifying it to the right degree. Of course we can breathe through our mouths, just as we can be fed through the nose or through the veins, but it is an emergency route and far inferior to the one which nature designed specifically for that purpose. In addition Yoga teaches that only the nose can extract the Prana present in the air. Lastly fresh air is naturally better than stale, and the air of the country, mountains or seaside is infinitely superior to that in cities.

Perhaps the reason for correct breathing being at the root of Hatha Yoga is because it is the quickest and soundest means by which we can control the emotions and the state of the mind. How many people who, feeling their temper rising, tell themselves to take a deep breath? Most nervous people find they can still their fears if they breathe slowly and deeply, and as one of the main objects of all Yoga is to control the mind, how better than by learning to master breathing?

Before beginning Pranayama it is as well to know a little elementary physiology of the chest. The lungs hang like twin balloons from just beneath the shoulders and when they are fully inflated, the diaphragm (a muscular floor separating the chest cavity from the abdominal cavity) is lowered to accommodate the distended lungs. It returns to its original place behind the ribs when the air is expelled and the lungs deflated. Although the working of the diaphragm is involuntary, like the heart, it can be operated deliberately, which the heart cannot. When the diaphragm is lowered, therefore, it increases the size of the chest and the lungs and when it relaxes, the chest and lungs contract as the air is expelled.

Yogis recognise three types of breathing:

1 Clavicular or upper breathing, practised by many people, is the worst and the most shallow breathing, named after the clavical (collar-bone). This uses only the smallest area of the lungs and it is common to many women who wear tight corsets, belts or other constrictions and to men who habitually sit in a slumped or hunched-up position, as when driving a car with a badly designed seat.

2 Mid- or intercostal breathing is slightly less inefficient than clavicular breathing, but not much.

The ribs are expanded slightly which may be nature's way of ensuring that man does not inhale too much stale air, for it is widely practised by people in crowded offices and factories.

3 Abdominal breathing is employed by most sleeping men and by others who have deliberately learnt it in the belief that it is better than the previous two, which it is. But it still falls far short of the type of breathing used instinctively by every animal and by primitive tribes.

It is obvious that a method of breathing which incorporates all the three types of breathing is to be preferred, and this is what is called the Complete Yoga Breath. It utilises the entire respiratory system, parts of which some people have not used since infancy, and it must be re-learnt systematically and slowly.

As with all Yoga exercises, this breathing exercise must be performed on an empty stomach in an airy room, or better still out-of-doors. Any clothing worn should be light and loose, and the bowels and bladder should have been emptied. The Lotus posture is ideal, but for novices this might be impossible. The closest approximation is to sit cross-legged, back upright, heels tucked in as close to the thighs as possible and the hands resting palms upwards on the knees, thumb and first fingertip lightly touching. This hand pose is called Jnana Mudra, a classic Yoga gesture, a symbol of true knowledge. The individual, respresented by the forefinger, is joined with the universe, represented by the thumb. The eyes should be closed to aid concentration.

The knees might stick up some distance from the floor to begin with, but as the hip-joints loosen, the knees will eventually lower and the posture becomes more comfortable. Those who find it quite impossible to sit cross-legged for more than a few minutes can stretch their legs out in front of them, but they are urged to attempt the correct posture daily until the muscles and joints are more flexible. It is not wise to sit in a chair because the success of Pranayama depends on the spine being kept in the correct position so as to support the lungs as they are exercised.

All breathing exercises begin by exhaling the breath to empty the lungs as completely as possible, and by slightly slumping the shoulders forward to aid this. No strain or force must be used. The facial and neck muscles should not be allowed to become tense and if it is found that too much effort is required, the exercise should be abandoned for the time being and tried again the next day. The essential is, if not comfort, relative ease.

Now, with the palm of the right hand placed lightly between the navel and the lower ribs, first exhale, then inhale, slowly and deeply, making the lung and abdomen expansion push out the hand.

Gradually slide the hand upwards until it lies between the nipples — in mid-chest — as more breath is taken in and this area expands too.

Lastly raise the shoulders very slightly, place the hand just below and between the collar bones as this part is filled with air.

Now reverse the procedure. Put the hand back on the abdomen. Don't push it in, but let it sink in naturally as the breath from that area is slowly released (through the nose, of course) and the hand follows the movement of the deflated lungs. Move the hand upwards and feel the same process as the breath is expelled from the middle chest, and further upwards as the rest of it is expelled from the upper parts of the lungs. It helps to imagine and visualise the lungs as balloons which expand when inflated and contract, fall flat, when deflated.

These movements must flow smoothly into one another without any jerkiness, but this may take time. For a few days it might be somewhat staccato, but after a week or so it should progress smoothly and by this time it should no longer be necessary to use the hands as guidelines. The lungs will have re-learnt their own work.

Repeat the movements slowly three times each day for a further week by which time it should never be forgotten. People who are uncertain of their progress in inflating successively the various parts of their lungs, should try doing the exercise in front of a large mirror, full face at first and then in profile. They will easily see the motions of their chest and abdominal muscles and if necessary can adjust their motions accordingly. Once you can control the inhalations and exhalations so that all three parts of the lungs are used, you can begin the Complete Yoga Breath, and in subsequent exercises the word 'breath' applies to the Complete Yoga Breath.

Sufferers from heart troubles, high blood pressure or detached retina must on no account retain the breath in, or hold it out, but may follow the directions for rhythmic Complete Yoga Breath.

EXERCISE I: THE COMPLETE YOGA BREATH

There is no part of the body which does not benefit from this exercise. It regulates the heartbeat, stimulates digestion and calms the nervous system. It has long been used by non-Yogic doctors and dentists who wanted to relieve their patients of tension resulting from intense pain during treatment, and public speakers and entertainers have used it to control nervousness. Mothers have been delivered of babies without anaesthetics by the use of whole breathing.

It is exactly the same as the preliminary exercise described above, except that each inhalation is made to the count of seconds or heartbeats.

1 Exhale — the first step in all Pranayama.

2 Inhale as slowly as possible, filling the lower lungs first as in the preliminary exercise, and going on to fill the middle and the upper lungs to the count you find most convenient. It might be 3, 5, 7 or 10 seconds.

3 Exhale slowly (this is difficult, the breath wants to gush out) to the same count as the inhalation without any jerkiness or pause. Remember, it must all be done through the nose and must be exhaled in the same order as (2) — first from the abdomen, second from the middle chest, and lastly from the upper chest.

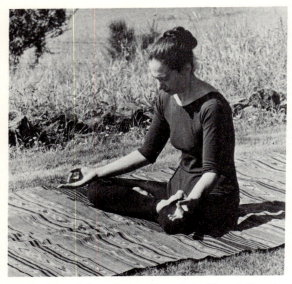

Complete exhalation (notice slumped shoulders, hollowed abdomen)

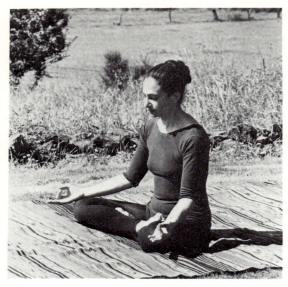

First stage of complete inhalation, abdomen filled with air

4 Slowly breathe in again and repeat from (2).

Perform the exercise three times in all, ending with an exhalation.

EXERCISE 2: KUMBHAKA

(The holding breath, a progression of Exercise 1).

1 Exhale.

2 Inhale slowly to a convenient count.

3 Hold in the breath for the same number of counts.

4 Exhale to the same number of counts.

5 Hold *out* the breath for the same number of counts.

Repeat the exercise three times.

Attention must be paid in this exercise to the tendency to gulp in air after having held the lungs empty for several seconds. If this is permitted, the lower lobes of the lungs are not filled with air and the amount inhaled is insufficient to inflate the total lung area. It is necessary to breathe in very slowly to allow all areas of the lungs to be inflated. Most students find it far more difficult to hold the breath *out* than *in*, and it is advisable to begin this exercise to a short count of three at the most. It cannot be stressed too often that no force must

ever be used in Yoga exercises. A mild discomfort is allowed but nothing more, and if strain is found to be necessary, it is harmful and it is *not* Yoga.

It is quite usual for an initial count of three seconds to build up to ten within a month. On the other hand people who smoke heavily often cannot achieve more than seven seconds. No

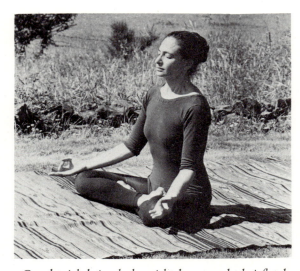

Complete inhalation, back upright, lungs completely inflated

matter, their lung expansion and oxygen intake will still be considerably improved and it has been noticed that smoking often becomes distasteful to those who have practised Pranayama for some weeks.

EXERCISE 3 : SUKH PURVAK
(Comfortable Pranayama)

Alternate nostril breathing in this exercise is recommended for sufferers from sinus and bronchial complaints. It soothes the nervous system and increases the powers of concentration.

1 Exhale.

2 Place the thumb of the right hand against the right nostril to close it, and let the first and second fingers of the same hand rest lightly on the centre of the forehead. Now breathe in slowly through the left nostril to a convenient count.

3 Remove the thumb from the right nostril and place the third, or ring-finger, of the right hand against the left nostril to close it.

4 Exhale through the right nostril to the same count as above.

5 Inhale through the right nostril to the same count.

6 Close the right nostril with the right thumb and exhale through the left nostril to the same count.

These six steps constitute one full cycle. Go back to (2) and repeat the procedure for three whole cycles in all.

EXERCISE 4

A progression from Exercise 3 is Exercise 4—similar, but with two differences. The breath is held into the lungs after each inhalation for the same length of time as the inhalation, and the lungs are held empty after each exhalation for the same time. Thus:

1 Exhale.

2 Inhale through left nostril, taking five seconds.

3 *Retain breath for five seconds.*

4 Exhale through right nostril for five seconds.

5 *Retain lungs empty for five seconds.*

6 Inhale through right nostril for five seconds.

7 *Retain breath in for five seconds.*

8 Exhale through left nostril for five seconds.

9 *Retain lungs empty for five seconds.*

This is one whole cycle. Repeat again from (2) until three complete cycles have been performed, making sure to end with (8) so that the exhalation is through the left nostril.

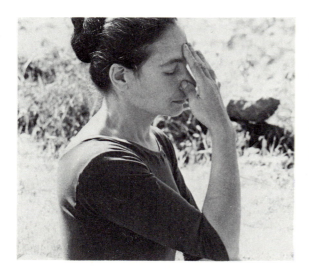
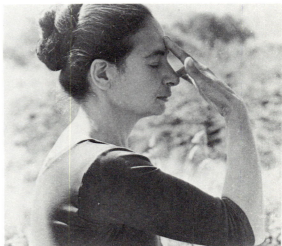

Alternate nostril breathing: Sukh Purvak

The last four exercises must not be attempted by people who, in addition to those who might suffer from high blood pressure, poor lungs and detached retina, have an over-active thyroid gland.

EXERCISE 5: UJJAYI OR CONQUEST

This stimulates the endocrine glands and particularly the thyroid. It raises abnormally low blood pressure and increases mental alertness.

1 Exhale.

2 Inhale slowly to the count of five to begin with.

3 Retain the breath for the same number of counts.

4 Expel the air *not* through the nostrils but by widening the mouth into a grin, top and bottom incisors touching as if biting a piece of cotton, making a 'ssss' sound, to a count *double* that of the inhalation — namely ten.

5 Inhale again without pause and repeat from (2).

It takes some practice to control the exhalation so that it does not start off in a good loud hiss only to falter and become weak and spasmodic towards the end. Similarly the hiss must not come in a series of jerks.

EXERCISE 6: KAPALABHATI OR THE CLEANSING BREATH

This is recommended for people who live in cities or who work in stuffy buildings. It helps those who find themselves in traffic jams or crowded rooms and who need to clear their lungs and nasal passages of smog, smoke or bacteria. It is advisable to blow the nose gently but thoroughly before beginning.

1 Exhale.

2 Inhale as deeply and as slowly as possible, to a convenient count.

3 Retain the breath for only *one* second.

4 Expel the air through the nostrils in a series of short, sharp blasts, as if blowing the nose only without a handkerchief. Make the exhalation take as long as possible, preferably not less than double the count of the inhalation and make the abdominal

muscles contract and relax in quick succession to force air out of the lungs.

Repeat from (2) without pause as soon as the lungs are quite empty, and repeat the whole exercise three times in all. As in Exercise 5, it takes practice before the exhalations maintain their vigour until the lungs are emptied.

EXERCISE 7:
(Progression of Exercise 5)

1 Exhale.

2 Inhale deeply and slowly to a convenient count.

3 Retain the breath for *one* second.

4 Exhale through the *mouth*, lips barely open, making a series of short, sharp 'ha ha' sounds for not less than double the count of the inhalation. It is not a continuous exhalation, but split up into emissions, and care must be taken that no air is inhaled in between emissions.

Repeat from (2), performing the whole exercise three times.

EXERCISE 8:
(Variation of Exercise 6)

1 Exhale.

2 Inhale deeply and slowly to a convenient count.

3 Retain the breath for *one* second.

4 Exhale the breath through the *mouth*, between clenched teeth in a series of short, sharp 'hiss' sounds. The front teeth should touch each other and the lips should be almost closed.

Repeat exercise three times in all.

EXERCISE 9: THE BELLOWS

This is a powerful exercise for removing toxins from the lungs and to help avoid infection. It relieves inflammation of the nasal passages and the throat, destroys phlegm, can help alleviate asthma and improves the circulation of the blood.

This exercise must not be done by people with detached retina or high blood pressure.

1 Exhale.

2 Inhale and exhale as quickly, deeply and as powerfully as possible (using the Complete Breath) in–out, in–out ten times.

3 Inhale the eleventh breath as slowly and as deeply as possible.

4 Retain the breath for 7–14 seconds.

5 Exhale slowly through the nose.

6 Without pausing, inhale again, repeating from (2).

Repeat three times in all.

The eyes should be kept closed when this exercise is first performed, for it is usual for some dizziness to be experienced. This is because air is reaching recesses of the lungs possibly for the first time. When this occurs, the exercise should be done just once in each session. When the dizziness disappears, as it will within a week or so, the eyes can be opened and the exercise be performed three times.

11 Loosening-up

Although extreme youth or age is no reason for preventing people to attempt Hatha Yoga, those who suffer from heart disease, high blood pressure or damaged joints should work only with an experienced teacher of therapeutic Yoga. Those who are overweight might find some difficulty in achieving sufficient flexibility to begin with, but as they progress the stimulation to the thyroid gland by some of the exercises should do much to reduce the weight and so remove the obstacle.

It is most important to remember that every movement must be made in slow motion and that force must never he used. Nor should pain be tolerated, although some discomfort should be expected when loosening-up or attempting a new exercise which may be using joints and muscles which are stiff with inaction.

Some of the asanas may seem impossible the first time of trying, but with daily practice the body regains the tone and loses its stiffness. Sometimes joints will creak alarmingly, but provided the exercises are attempted gently and slowly, no harm will result. It will be easier if the student can set aside a regular half hour or more every day, and morning is preferable. It is easier to perform the exercises later in the day when the body has become more supple, but progress will be quicker if they are done early, despite the initial difficulty.

Choose a well-ventilated room or a private garden, wear as few clothes as possible, or in the privacy of your own room, be naked. In any event there must be no constrictions or tight bands at throat, chest, waist or arms. The feet should be bare.

Arm-circling exercises (showing left arm)

Each student should have his own rug or mat on which to perform, and it should be of the non-slip variety — a thick cotton mat is often less slippery than wool. It is not advisable to use foam rubber for it upsets the sense of balance in certain poses. Yoga teachers maintain that by always using the same mat we develop an affinity with it, so that it helps us to induce the right state of mind. Hygiene is a more mundane, but none the less valid, reason since the mouth and the nose are frequently pressed into the mat, making cleanliness an essential.

Yoga must be done on an empty — or at least unfilled — stomach which has had no food or drink for the previous two hours. Similarly the

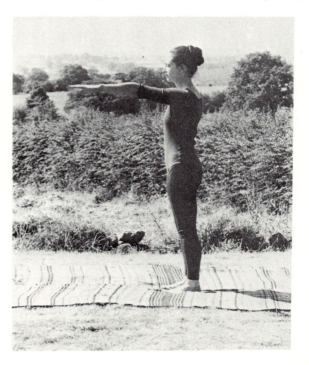

bladder should be emptied or discomfort might be felt. Start by relaxing for at least ten minutes. The next ten minutes are spent on breathing exercises, and last of all the Yoga asanas. For the first week or two the student must concentrate on working the stiffness of years out of his body. Those who engage in sports activities regularly find that only a few of the less-used muscles and joints need attention, but for most people every part of the body will have to be dealt with before the asanas can be attempted.

Although many callisthenics can be used to loosen up, the following are specifically arranged to prepare the body for Yoga exercises.

EXERCISE I: FORWARD ARM CIRCLING

1 Stand erect, arms at side, feet about 9in apart.

2 Slowly raise the right arm forward to shoulder level.

3 Continue raising the arm, elbow remaining stiff, directly overhead, letting it touch the ear as it passes, and lower it backwards until it drops back to the side. The arm actually rotates in its socket when the elbow is kept stiff and kept close to the ear as it passes overhead.

Repeat three times with each arm.

EXERCISE 2: BACKWARD ARM CIRCLING

1 Stand erect, arms at sides, feet about 9in apart.

2 Raise the right arm straight in front up to chest level.

3 Lower it slowly down, past the hips, touching them as it does so. Rotate the shoulder in the socket, elbow remaining stiff, the arm brushing past the ear as it passes overhead to the front of the body and then dropping relaxed to the side.

Repeat from (2) three times with the right arm and three times with the left.

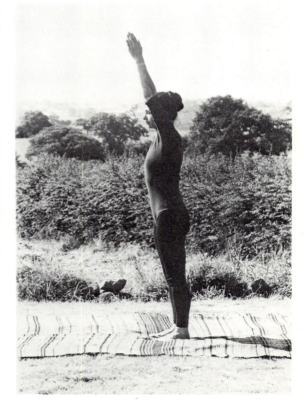

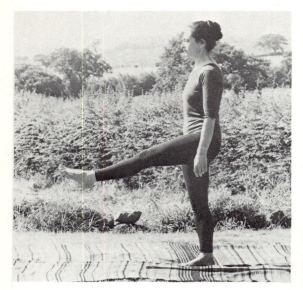

resisted. Hold the position for a few moments.

3 Slowly swing the leg down and backwards so that the foot just touches the floor and the leg brushes the other knee and passes it without pause and goes backwards as high as it can. Again keep the trunk erect and both knees stiff. Hold the position for a few moments.

4 Slowly lower the leg to the ground.

Repeat three times with each leg. This exercise has the dual purpose of loosening-up the hips and waist and developing a sense of balance essential for many Yoga exercises.

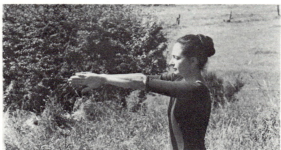

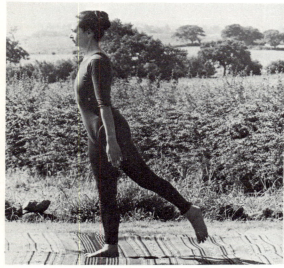

Leg-swinging exercises

EXERCISE 3: LEG SWINGING

1 Stand erect, arms by the sides, feet about 9in apart.

2 Keeping the knees stiff, slowly raise the left leg in front as high as possible. The trunk should remain upright and the tendency to counter-balance the body by leaning back must be

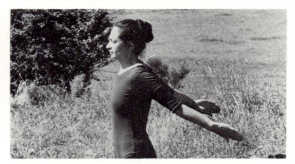

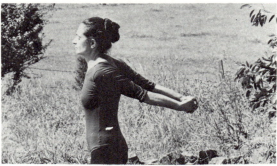

Hand-clapping exercises

EXERCISE 4: HAND CLAPPING

1 Standing erect, feet about 9in apart, slowly raise both arms (elbows stiff) forward to chest level and turn backs of hands together.

2 Inhale as the arms are slowly moved round, outwards and backwards at chest level (as if doing the breast-stroke in swimming) until the palms can be clapped behind the back. The elbows will probably bend at first before the hands touch, but they should be kept as stiff as possible and the trunk should be erect.

3 Holding the breath, clasp the fingers tight and try to raise the joined hands high behind the shoulders, stiffening the elbows in doing so and keeping the trunk erect.

4 Slowly exhale as the hands are released and the arms are lowered to the sides.

Repeat three times.

EXERCISE 5: HEAD TURNING

1 Stand erect with feet about 9in apart, arms by the sides.

2 Slowly turn the head to the left as far as possible. Pause.

3 Slowly bring the head to the front and, without pause, turn it as far to the right as possible. Pause.

4 Slowly bring the head back until looking straight ahead.

Repeat three times.

At first considerable creaking might be heard and felt at the back of the neck during this and the following neck exercises, but so long as no force is used and no jerkiness permitted, it is of no concern. It is due to the great amount of tension which most of us develop in the nape of the neck, and within two or three weeks the sounds should diminish and the neck move more freely.

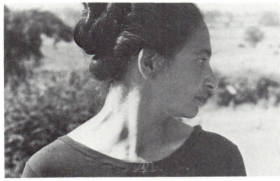

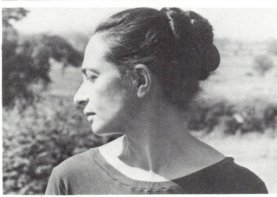

Head-turning exercises (both stages)

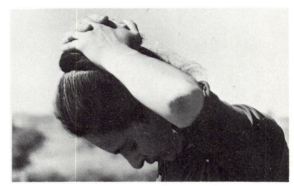

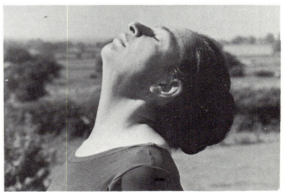

Head-nodding exercises (both stages)

EXERCISE 6: HEAD NODDING

1 Stand erect, feet about 9in apart, arms by the sides.

2 Slowly lower the head to press the chin against the chest, making sure that the shoulders do not move.

3 Place both hands on the crown of the head and press it gently down as far as it will go, the chin digging into the chest.

4 Remove the hands and slowly raise the head, letting it hang behind as far as possible.

5 Now open the mouth wide for a second before closing it. Increased tightness will then be felt under the chin as the neck is stretched.

6 Slowly lower the head to its original position. Repeat three times.

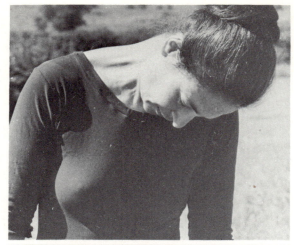

EXERCISE 7: HEAD ROLLING

1 Stand erect with feet about 9in apart, arms by the sides.

2 Resisting any tendency to raise the shoulders, slowly lower the head until the chin touches the chest.

3 In a continuous, slow movement, rotate the head to the left, so that it lolls on the left shoulder, lolls backwards above the spine and then lolls on to the right shoulder and so to the front until it flops on to the chest.

4 Repeat from (2) but in the opposite direction, that is, rotating the head to the right.

This exercise should be done three times in each direction, six rotations in all.

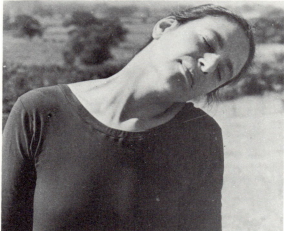

The three neck exercises are among the most important Yoga exercises, not only because they are a quick and reliable means of instantly removing tension, but also because nearly every Yoga exercise incorporates the neck, and it is necessary to have it flexible before beginning the asanas. They can be done sitting as well as standing.

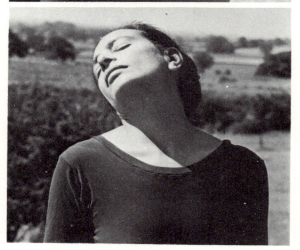

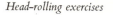

Head-rolling exercises

EXERCISE 8: PADAHASTASANA OR THE STORK
(Bending and stretching)

This is a Yoga asana — a classical pose — and it is an excellent method of loosening the muscles.

1 Stand erect with the feet together, arms by the sides.

2 Inhale and slowly raise the arms, elbows stiff, above the head.

3 Exhale and slowly lower the arms and trunk, keeping the knees stiff throughout.

4 Grasp the ankles, widen the bent elbows and place the head as near as possible to the knees. Hold the pose for several seconds.

5 Inhale as you slowly straighten the trunk keeping the arms relaxed and hanging loose, and return to (1).

Repeat three times.

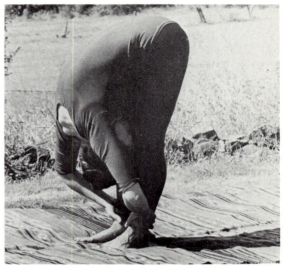

Padahastasana: the Stork, stretching and bending

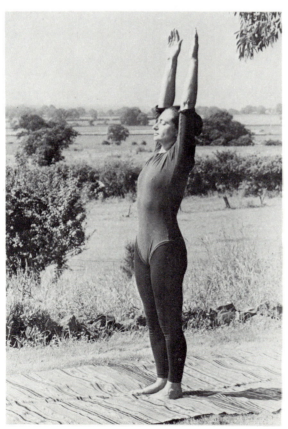

It is quite likely that many people will not be able to reach their ankles, let alone grasp them, and considerable stiffness will subsequently be felt at the back of the thighs. Nevertheless even elderly and obese students have achieved the pose after a few weeks of daily practice, and it is invaluable in making parts of the body flexible in preparation for more advanced asanas.

EXERCISE 9: HIP LOOSENING

1 Sit on the floor with both legs outstretched in front, touching each other, knees stiff.

2 Slowly bend the right knee, keeping the lower leg vertical, the sole of the foot flat on the floor and touching the other leg, and bring the heel as close as possible to the right thigh, the foot remaining parallel to the left leg.

3 With the left hand, hold the right foot in position.

4 Put the right hand on the right knee.

5 Gently and slowly push the right knee outwards and down towards the floor as much as possible and at the same time allow the sole of the right foot to lie against the inside of the left thigh, the left

hand making sure that the heel remains tucked into the crotch.

6 Raise the right knee back to (2).

Repeat three times with each leg.

It is imperative that no force is used in pushing the knees towards the ground, only the gentlest pressure must be applied. In the beginning some people can achieve little more than a few inches movement, but progress is rapid.

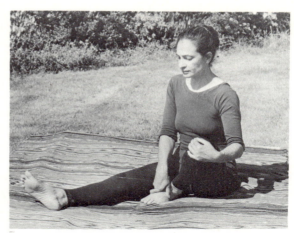

Ankle loosening, second stage

2 Slowly bend the right knee, keeping the lower leg vertical, the sole of the foot flat on the floor and touching the other leg, and bring the heel as close as possible to the right thigh, the foot being parallel to the left leg.

3 With the left hand, hold the foot in position.

4 With the right hand, gently push the knee to the right as far as possible, but keep the sole of the right foot flat on the floor throughout, held in position by the left hand so that the ankle is being flexed.

5 Bring the knee upwards to (2).

Repeat three times with each leg.

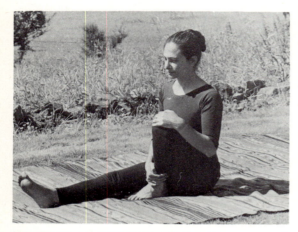

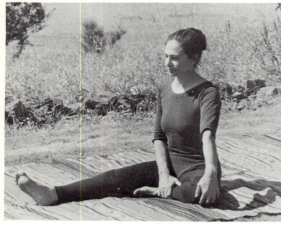

Hip loosening, both stages (showing left leg)

EXERCISE 10: ANKLE LOOSENING

1 Sit upright with both legs outstretched in front, touching each other and knees stiff.

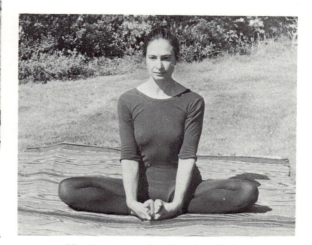

Baddha Konasana: pelvic loosening, final stage

EXERCISE 11: BADDHA KONASANA
(Pelvic loosening)

1 Sit erect, legs outstretched, touching each other.

2 Slowly bend the knees as wide apart as possible to bring the soles of the feet together and as close to the body as possible.

3 Interlace the fingers of both hands and cradle the toes, drawing them nearer to the body.

4 Slowly and gently widen the knees and get them as close to the ground as possible. Pause for a few seconds.

5 Slowly return to (1).

Repeat three times.

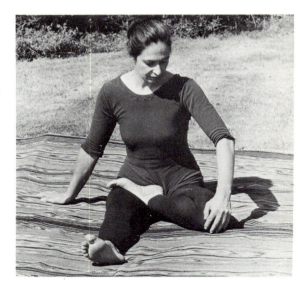

EXERCISE 12: LOOSENING FOR THE LOTUS POSE

1 Sit erect with legs outstretched in front, touching each other.

2 Clasp the left ankle with the right hand so that the thumb is on the inside of the ankle pointing towards the floor.

3 Slowly lift the left ankle as high as possible, bending the left knee and carry it on to the right thigh as close to the groin as possible.

4 Lower the left knee as near to the ground as possible, keeping the right leg stiff. Hold for a few seconds.

5 Still using the right hand, lift the left foot from the groin and take it back to the position in (2), straightening the knee on the way.

6 Return to (1).

Repeat three times with each leg.

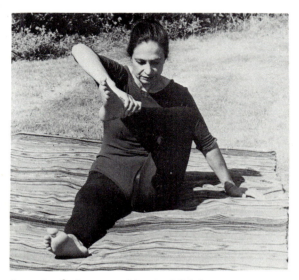

Loosening for Lotus pose (showing left leg)

EXERCISE 13: FURTHER LOTUS LOOSENING

1 Sit erect with legs outstretched touching each other.

2 With the right hand, grasp the right ankle, bending the knee outwards towards the floor, and slide the outer edge of the foot along the floor until the sole lies against the inner right thigh close to the crotch.

3 With the left hand, grasp the left ankle and repeat the same action as in (2), bringing the left heel in front of (but not on top of) the right ankle. The feet will then lie beside each other, both outer edges touching the floor and both knees as close to the floor as possible.

4 Using both hands, lift the left foot on top of the right foot, one heel on top of the other.

5 Using both hands, lift the left foot further up to the right thigh, keeping the left knee close to the ground. Pause.

6 Using both hands, lift the left foot from the thigh and replace it back on top of the other foot as in (4).

7 With both hands, lift the left foot off the other and lay it beside the right foot as in (3).

8 Remove the hands and slowly straighten out the legs until they are in the position indicated in (1).

Repeat the exercise three times with each leg.

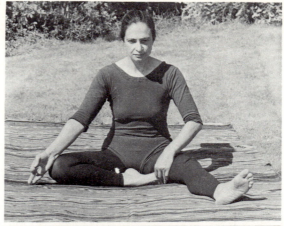

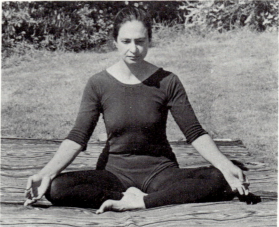

Further loosening exercises for the Lotus pose on this and facing page

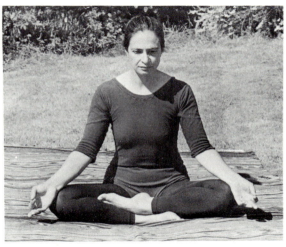

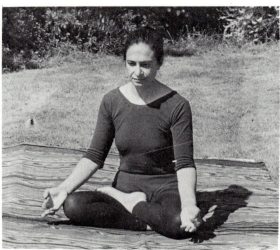

Although most of the loosening-up exercises can be abandoned once some flexibility is achieved and the Yoga asanas have begun, the following must be continued at frequent intervals throughout the practice of Hatha Yoga: Exercises 5, 6, 7 (head and neck), 8 (the Stork) and 11 (Baddha Konasana). Exercises 11, 12 and 13 can be discontinued when the Lotus pose is perfected.

Every Yoga session, including the loosening-up exercises, ends as it begins, with complete relaxation. The suggested times must, of necessity, be adapted to suit the person but whatever else has to be curtailed, the relaxation is essential and must not be omitted. It can, if necessary, be shortened but experienced Yogis claim that the full benefit cannot be gained unless at least ten minutes are spent in the Savasana or Dead pose. Others maintain that at least half an hour should be devoted to relaxation at least one day a week, even if on that day there is no time for other exercises. It is up to the individual to decide once he learns which benefits him most.

12   Yoga Asanas or Exercises

Each of the Yoga asanas or poses has been developed over the centuries to benefit various parts or organs of the body, and students practising Hatha Yoga without a teacher are advised to learn them in the order given in this book, since proficiency in one helps to prepare the body for the next. Some are easier to achieve than others, and when they can all be performed the student can choose those which might help his physical condition. Each must be done very slowly with no force.

SARVANGASANA: THE SHOULDER STAND OR CANDLE

This is one of the most beneficial exercises for the entire body. By the pressure it exerts on the thyroid gland in the base of the neck, it causes an increased flow of blood to that area and helps to regulate its malfunction. The inverted position benefits sufferers

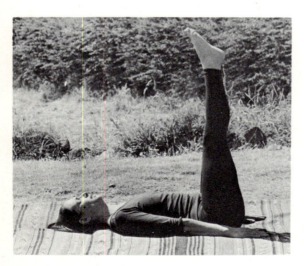

Sarvangasana: the Shoulder Stand or Candle, first stage

from asthma, bronchitis and throat complaints and affects the abdomen so that constipation, menstrual troubles, urinary disorders and piles gain relief. The mind must dwell on the thyroid gland throughout the exercise.

Warning: people with high blood pressure should not attempt this asana until they can perform the Plough (next asana) and hold that pose for three minutes.

First stage

1 Lie in the Dead pose.
2 Exhale and at the same time very slowly raise both legs keeping the knees stiff until they are at right angles to the body, the toes pointing upwards.
3 Pause for a moment, inhale then exhale.
4 Inhale and at the same time slowly lower the legs to the ground, keeping them close together and stiff.
5 Pause and repeat the exercise three times in all. The slower this can be performed the more benefit it brings to the abdominal muscles.

Second stage

Follow the previous steps up to (3) when the legs are at right-angles to the body.

4 Press the palms of the hands on the floor beside the body and at the same time raise the buttocks from the floor and bring the legs up — knees stiff — until they are angled over the head, the toes pointing.
5 Bend the arms and place the hands behind the waist to support the hips, so that the weight of the body is taken by the arms. Pause for a few seconds.
6 Remove the hands and slowly straighten the arms on to the floor so that the palms take the weight of the body.

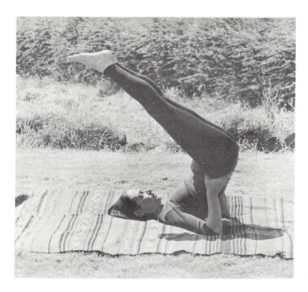

The Shoulder Stand, second stage

the arms to the floor and let the palms take the weight.

10 Slowly lower the buttocks until the legs are at right angles to the body.

11 Slowly lower the legs until they are on the ground and the body is in the Dead pose. There is a tendency for the head to pop up as the stiff legs are almost on the ground, and this must be resisted.

12 The Dead pose must be maintained for the same time that the body was in a vertical position, otherwise dizziness will occur.

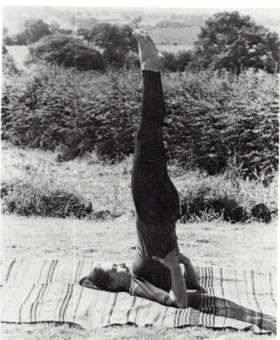

The Shoulder Stand, third stage

7 Slowly lower the buttocks until the legs are vertical as in (3).

8 Slowly lower the legs to the ground as in (1).

Third stage

Repeat the previous steps to (5) when the hands will be supporting the body and the straight legs angled over the head.

6 Tuck in the buttocks, slowly straighten the spine, shifting the hands higher up the back to the shoulder blades, and at the same time bringing the legs vertical, knees stiff, the toes relaxed and the chin pressed very hard into the chest. It should be almost impossible to speak at this point, and the body should be in a vertical line from the feet to the shoulders.

7 Breathe abdominally and stay in the pose for as long as possible, beginners starting with a few seconds and eventually maintaining it for up to ten minutes.

8 Slowly lower the hands until they are behind the waist and the legs are angled over the head as in (5).

9 Remove the hands from the waist, straighten

SHOULDER STAND: VARIATION I

When vertical in the shoulder stand, slowly remove the arms from the ground and bring them to rest against the side so that the fingers are pointing upwards towards the feet. It may take some time before the balance is perfected and the pose can be sustained with the hands thus.

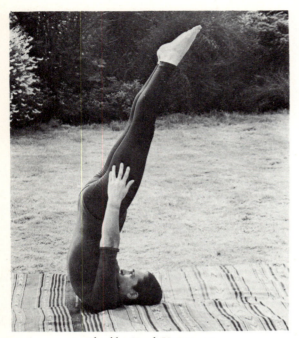

Shoulder Stand, Variation 1

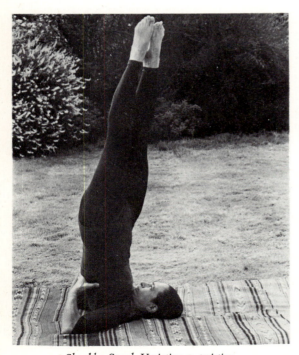

Shoulder Stand, Variation 2, twisting

SHOULDER STAND: VARIATION 2

When vertical in the shoulder stand, the hands supporting the upper shoulder-blades, slowly and gently twist the lower trunk and legs to the right as far as they will go. Hold the pose for a few moments, return to the central position, and then slowly turn to the left.

HALASANA: THE PLOUGH

This is particularly good for people suffering from lumbago, liver and kidney troubles. Like the shoulder stand, it increases the flow of blood to the thyroid gland and helps to regulate obesity, especially round the hips. It releases pressure and compression on the vertebrae, making the spine more flexible and often removing the cause of headaches.

Warning: no upside-down pose should be practised during menstruation.

1 Lie flat on the floor in the Dead pose.

2 Slowly raise the stiff legs until at right angles to the body, toes pointing upwards.

3 Press the palms of the hands on the floor and at the same time raise the buttocks and bring the legs up, still stiff, until they are angled over the head, the toes pointing.

4 Bend the arms and support the hips by placing the hands behind the waist, so that the arms take the weight. Pause a few seconds.

5 Tuck in the buttocks, slowly straighten the spine, shifting the hands towards the shoulder-blades and at the same time bringing the legs vertical and the body in a straight line, chin pressed against the chest.

6 Slowly bring one leg over the head until the toes touch the ground, keeping the other leg vertical. Both must remain stiff.

7 Perform this scissor-like action slowly three times with each leg.

8 Slowly lower both legs to the ground over the head, toes turned under and their tips pointing towards the head, and at the same time lower the

arms flat on the ground, palms downward, in the opposite direction to the legs. Pause for a few seconds.

9 Now point the toes further away from the head so that the toenails are touching the floor and the spine is curved even more, and the chin pressed even tighter against the chest.

10 Slowly bring the hands up and, with the fingers, touch first the ears and then the toes, repeating the movement three times. The arms must slide along the floor and not lose contact with it.

11 Stretch the arms along the floor above the head, fingers pointing towards the toes. Hold the pose for as long as possible, increasing the time to five minutes when fully proficient.

12 Slowly bring the hands behind the waist to take the weight.

13 Avoiding jerkiness, uncoil the spine and bring the legs up angled over the head keeping the knees stiff throughout.

14 Remove hands from the back and lay them

palm downwards on the floor to take the weight.

15 Slowly lower the buttocks to the floor, bringing the legs up vertical and at right angles to the body. Pause.

16 Slowly lower legs to the floor, into the Dead pose. To avoid dizziness, this position must be held for as long as the body was inverted.

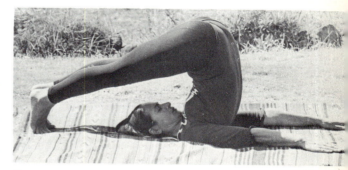

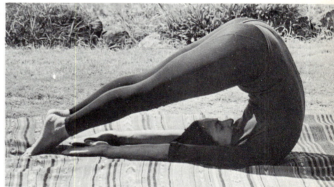

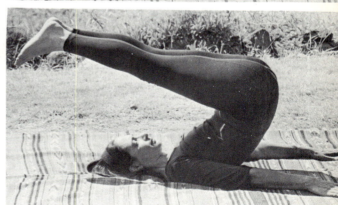

Halasana: the Plough, successive stages

MATSYASANA: THE FISH

This pose is dedicated to the fish which was the incarnation of Vishnu and which was supposed, at the time of the flood, to have warned the Hindu Adam of the forthcoming disaster.

It is good for infected tonsils and for head colds, it relieves inflamed piles and has a beneficial effect on the thyroid gland. It is on the thyroid that the student should concentrate while performing it.

First stage

This is for students who cannot perform the Lotus pose.

1 Sit erect, legs outstretched in front, side by side.

2 Place the hands on the hips, by the waist.

3 Slowly lower each elbow on the floor behind the body until the elbows are supporting the trunk.

4 Arch the spine into as deep a hollow as possible, throwing back the head in a continuous curve until the crown of the head is on the floor and the elbows wider apart. If this is not achieved, carefully remove one hand from the waist and use it to push the forehead gently to increase the curve of the spine.

5 Remove both hands and place them lightly on the abdomen so that the weight of the body is taken by the head and the buttocks. Make sure that the mouth is kept closed. Hold for up to one minute.

6 Slowly slide the head until the spine is on the floor and the body has returned to (1).

Second stage

1 Sit in the Lotus pose.

2 Place hands on hips by the waist.

3 Slowly lower each elbow to the floor behind the body until they are supporting the trunk.

4 Arch the spine, throw back the head until the crown is on the floor, the elbows wider apart and the back arched as much as possible.

5 With the right hand grasp the left toes, and with the left hand the right toes, removing the elbows from the ground.

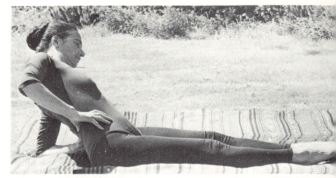
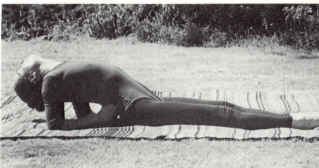
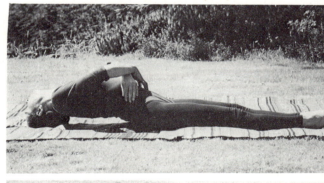
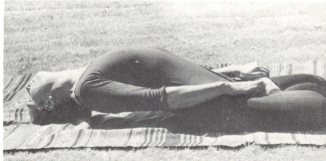

Matsyasana: the Fish, both variations

6 Gently increase the arch of the spine by pulling on the toes.

7 Hold for up to one minute, breathing as deeply as possible.

8 Let go of the toes, uncurl the legs and slide the head until the body has assumed the Dead pose.

Relax for a few moments before repeating the exercise with the legs crossed the other way in the Lotus (ie, if the right leg was bent first during the first exercise, begin the second with the left one bent first).

When both have been done, lie in the Dead pose for three minutes before sitting up.

PASCHIMOTTANASANA: STRETCHING

This is particularly good for the heart since it increases peristaltic action. The slow stretching of the back makes the spine more supple, tones the sciatic nerve and can cure impotence.

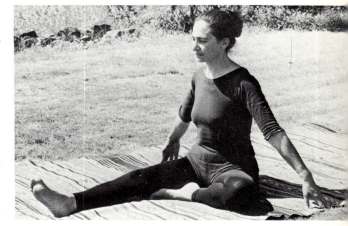

First stage

This is a complete exercise in itself.

1 Sit erect on floor, legs outstretched in front, arms out sideways with the fingertips touching the floor.

2 Bend the right leg until the sole of the foot is alongside the inner left thigh, the heel as close to the crotch as possible and the right knee as close to the floor as possible. The left leg must remain stiff.

3 Exhale and inhale immediately.

4 Exhale and stretch both arms towards the left foot, clasping the fingers around the instep, bringing the head to touch the knees and keeping the elbows wide apart and up from the floor.

5 Pause for a few seconds, increasing the time up to three minutes, breathing normally.

6 Exhale, inhale and return to (2) with the left leg outstretched, the right sole against the left inner thigh and the fingertips touching the floor at either side of the body.

Repeat three times with each leg.

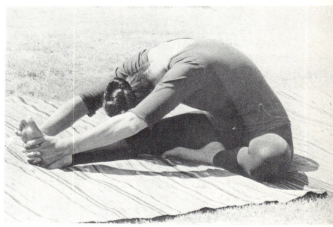

Paschimottanasana: stretching, first stage (showing left leg)

Second stage

1 Sit erect, legs outstretched in front, arms out sideways with fingertips touching the floor.

2 Exhale and inhale immediately.

3 Exhale and at the same time stretch forward until each hand grasps the respective ankle — the thumb uppermost, the elbows and forearms on the floor alongside the legs and the head touching the knee.

4 Hold the pose for as long as possible, starting with a few seconds and extending up to three minutes.

5 Inhale as you remove the hands, straighten the back and return to (1).

Pause and repeat three times with each leg.

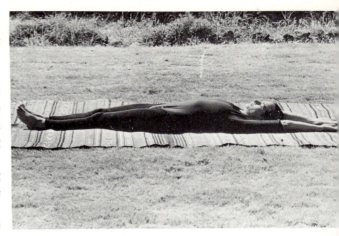

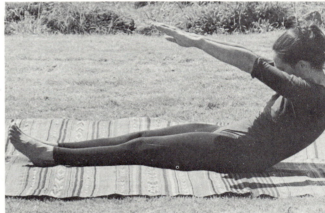

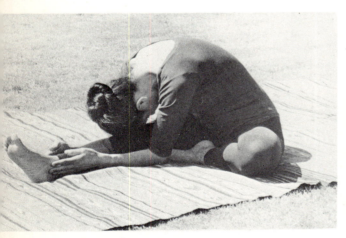

Paschimottanasana: stretching, second stage

Third stage

1 Lie in the Dead pose.

2 Exhale.

3 Inhale and sweep the straightened arms overhead until they are on the floor.

4 Exhale and at the same time raise the arms and the upper trunk, curling the spine forwards until the hands clasp the respective ankles, thumb uppermost, the elbows and forearms are on the floor and the head on the knees.

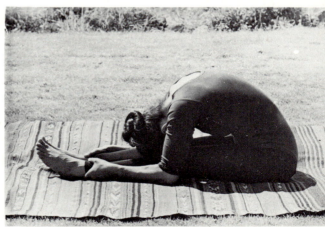

Paschimottanasana: stretching, third stage

5 Hold the pose for up to three minutes.

6 Slowly inhale as you come out of the pose, straighten the back and let the hands slide up the legs and return to the Dead pose as in (1).

Relax for a few moments before repeating the exercise three times in all.

Note: there is a tendency for the feet to pop up as the upper trunk and arms are raised in (4). If this persists, either have somebody lightly push down the feet at this step or put the feet under a piece of furniture such as a settee until proficiency is achieved. This is, of course, only a temporary aid.

Fourth stage

1 Sit erect, legs outstretched in front, arms outstretched at sides with fingertips touching the floor.

2 Exhale.

3 Inhale and curl the toes towards the face.

4 Exhale and reach down until each palm cradles the toes and sole of the foot. Ideally the toes should rest on the inner wrist but to begin with the fingers may only just reach the toes.

5 Inhale and stretch the body upwards, throwing back the head and hollowing the back, making sure that the knees are kept absolutely stiff and flat on the ground.

6 Exhale and look down, bringing the head in line with the arms.

7 Inhale and slowly remove the hands and return to (1).

Pause and perform three or more times.

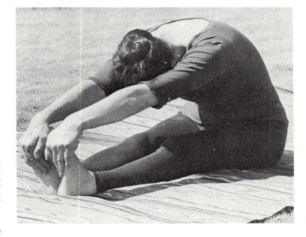

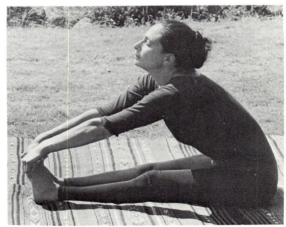

Paschimottanasana: stretching fourth stage

PADAHASTASANA: THE STORK

This is a stretching exercise with benefits similar to those in the previous exercise, but as the head is held low, the effect on the brain is intensified. It improves memory and benefits the sinuses. It is a variation of the leg-stretching exercise described in Chapter 11.

1 Stand erect, feet close together, arms by side, and exhale.

2 Inhale and at the same time raise both arms forward until they are directly overhead.

3 Exhale as you bend down, keeping arms over the head, until the fingers are under the feet, the toes resting on the wrists and only the heels on the floor. The knees must remain stiff.

4 Inhale and look up, hollowing the back as much as possible, pushing the buttocks back to increase the arch of the spine. Bring the head as far back as possible.

5 Exhale and look down.

6 Inhale and let hands fall and slide up the legs until the body is upright as in (1).

Note: in the beginning perhaps only the fingers will be under the feet and can only just clasp the toes. Practice will improve this.

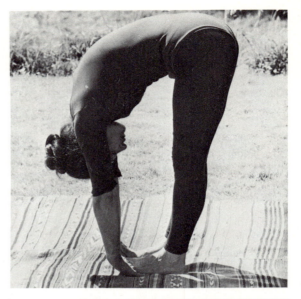

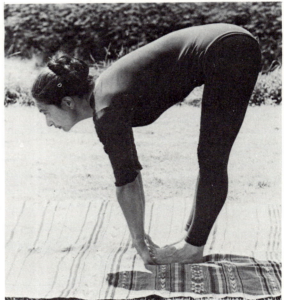

Padahastasana: the Stork, variation

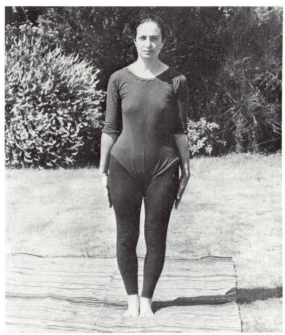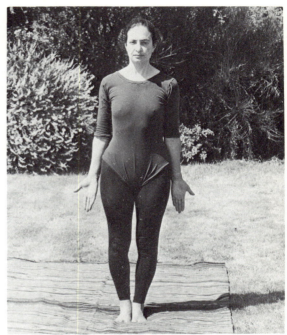

Tadasana: the Mountain, both stages

TADASANA: THE MOUNTAIN

This is a symbolic exercise of Yoga, the one step when the body is receptive, the other when it is inward looking. In addition it is an important means of acquiring poise and correct body balance. It has the advantage of being far less strenuous than most poses and can therefore be performed by almost everyone.

1 Stand erect, feet touching along their whole length and the toes stretched flat out on the floor. The arms hang by the sides, the knees must be pushed hard back so that the legs are rigid and the kneecaps pulled upwards and inwards. The weight must be distributed evenly all over the feet, neither on just the heel nor just the toes. The arms are stiff, head and shoulders erect.

2 Exhale.

3 Inhale and at the same time slowly rotate the forearms until the palms are facing forwards, the biceps will be turned forwards by the action and it should be felt in the shoulders which will immediately become straighter. The elbows must remain against the sides and quite stiff.

4 Exhale and return to (1).

Repeat several times.

VRKSASANA: THE TREE, FIRST POSE

This exercise tones the leg muscles and helps the student to develop a sense of balance. For those with poor balance, it is best to fix the eyes on a stationary object until poise is gained.

1 Stand erect, feet touching along their whole length and the toes stretched out flat on the floor. Stiffen arms and place by the sides. Push knees back hard so that the legs are rigid and the kneecaps pulled upwards and inwards. The weight must be distributed evenly over all the feet. Head and shoulders erect.

2 Slowly bend the right leg and bring the foot up until the hand can grasp it. Do not bend the body or the balance will be lost. Place the right heel firmly into the crotch so that the sole of the right foot, toes pointing downwards, is resting against the inner left thigh.

3 Balance on the left leg while you slowly place hands palms together at waist level and slowly raise them directly overhead as high as possible.

4 Stretch, fingers pointing upwards and maintaining the balance.

5 Hold the pose for a few seconds.

6 Slowly lower hands and right leg and regain position in (1).

Repeat once with the other leg.

Note: it is important to obey every step exactly: unless (1) is perfectly performed, the rest cannot succeed.

VRKSASANA: THE TREE, SECOND POSE

1 Stand erect as in (1) of the first Tree pose.

2 Raise the right foot, using both hands and keeping body erect until the right foot lies on the

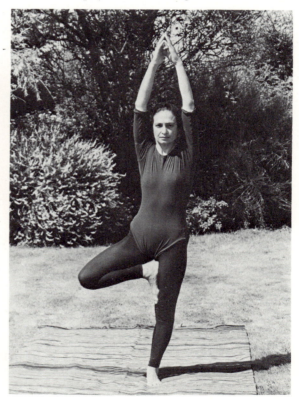

Vrksasana: the Tree, three variations each with two stages

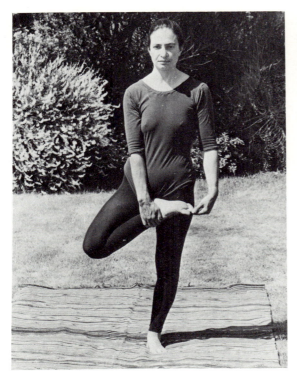

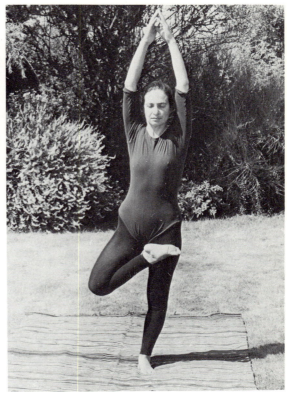

left thigh as high as possible, sole facing upwards and the right knee pointing outwards and *not* forwards.

3 Once the balance is achieved, slowly remove the hands.

4 Place the palms together at waist level and slowly raise arms overhead.

5 Hold the pose for a few seconds.

6 Slowly lower the hands and the leg, regaining (1). Repeat with the other leg.

VRKSASANA: THE TREE, THIRD POSE

Warning: do not attempt this until the previous Tree poses have been perfected. People with bad knees or a history of cartilage troubles should not attempt this pose.

1 Stand erect as in (1) of the previous Tree poses.

2 Raise the right leg and, helped by the hands, bring the right foot on to the left hip, so that the

upper part of the right leg — the thigh — is parallel to that of the left leg. The sole should face upwards and the knees should be alongside each other.

3 When balance is achieved, slowly remove the hands and bend the elbows, keeping them touching the waist until the forearms are parallel with the floor and facing forwards, and the palms are facing upwards.

4 Hold the pose for a few seconds.

5 Slowly lower the arms and the leg until (1) is reached. Pause and repeat with the other leg.

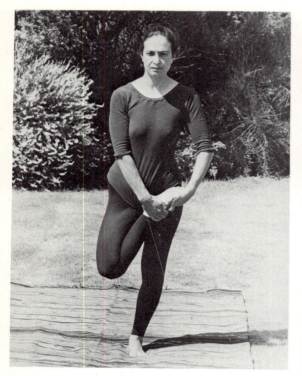
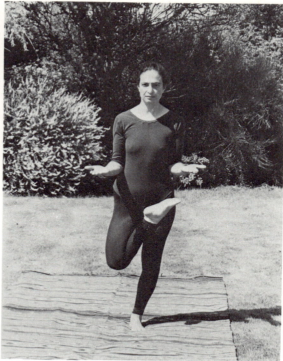

Vrksasana: the Tree, third pose

SALABHASANA: THE LOCUST OR GRASSHOPPER

So named because the pose is similar to that of the grasshopper resting on the ground. The bladder and, in men, the prostate gland benefit, as do those suffering from flatulence or gastric troubles. In addition it helps those who have pain in the sacral or lumbar regions.

First stage

1 Lie face down on floor with nose and forehead touching the floor. *Note:* if preferred, the chin alone can rest on the floor.

2 Make fists of the hands, with thumb and forefinger pressing on the floor.

3 Exhale.

4 Inhale and at the same time raise the right leg, keeping the knee stiff and pushing down on the fists so that the right hip is slightly raised from the floor.

5 Hold pose for a few seconds.

6 Lower leg to the floor.

7 Pause and repeat three times with each leg in scissor movement.

Second stage

1 Lie face down on the floor as in (1) in the previous asana.

2 Either make fists of the hands or place them palm against the front of the thighs, backs of hand pressing hard against the floor, fingers pointed towards feet.

3 Exhale.

4 Inhale and lift both feet and legs off the floor, keeping knees absolutely stiff, and raise the legs as close together as possible and as high as possible, pressing down hard with either the backs of the

hands or the fists against the floor, the weight being borne by the hands, arms, and the head.

Hold for a few seconds.

Note: for a few days the legs may rise only an inch or even less.

Third stage

1 Lie face down on floor as in (1) in the previous two asanas.

2 Let hands lie by the sides, palms upwards.

3 Exhale.

4 Inhale and at the same time raise the upper trunk, the legs stiff and the arms stiff, all being raised as high as possible.

5 Hold the pose for a few moments, increasing if possible.

6 Exhale and relax, returning to position at (2).

7 Relax for a few moments.

Repeat three times.

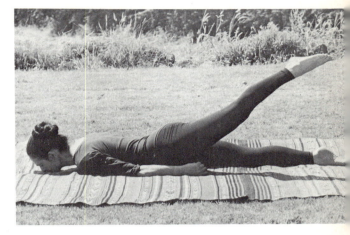

BHUJANGASANA: THE COBRA

In India this asana is performed to prevent the formation of kidney stones. Here it prevents fatty tissues forming on hips. In addition it increases flexibility of the spine and expands the chest.

1 Lie flat on the floor, face downwards.

2 Place the palms on the floor by the sides of the shoulders, the fingertips level with the shoulders and pointing towards the head.

3 Exhale.

4 Inhale, and without putting any pressure on the hands, raise the upper trunk, the head thrown back to increase the hollow in the spine.

5 Now, putting slight pressure on the hands, raise the trunk even higher, making sure that the navel remains in contact with the floor so that the elbows remain bent, shoulders back.

6 Hold the pose for a few seconds.

7 Exhale as you slowly return to the floor and resume position at (2).

8 Relax for a few moments.

Repeat three times.

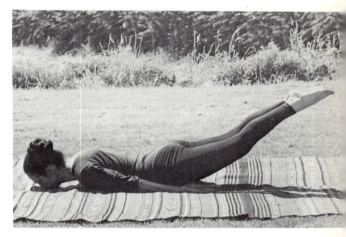

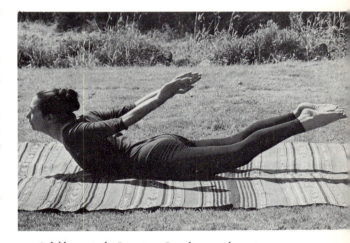

Salabhasana: the Locust or Grasshopper, three stages

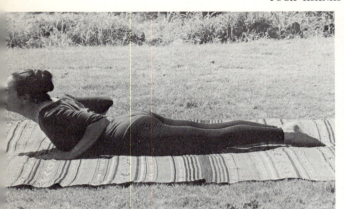
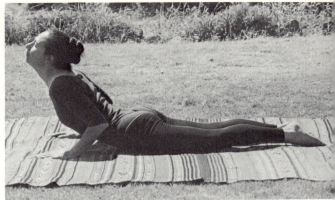

Bhujangasana: the Cobra, both stages

URDHVA MUKHA SVANASANA: THE DOG

Those suffering from a stiff back, lumbago, sciatica and from slipped or prolapsed discs of the spine benefit from this. The lungs gain elasticity and the pelvic region is aided.

1 Lie flat on the floor, face down.

2 Point the toes so that the soles face the ceiling. The feet should be about 1ft apart.

3 Place the palms of the hands on the floor at waist level, fingers pointing towards the head.

4 Exhale.

5 Inhale and raise the head and upper trunk, putting the full weight on the palms until the arms are stiff. Throw back the head, look towards the ceiling and throw out the chest.

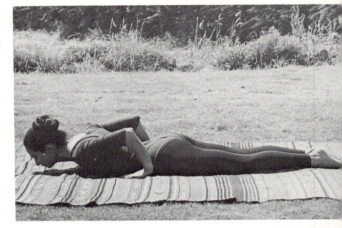

6 The weight must be on the hands and the upper toes only, the legs must remain stiff and the knees just off the ground, so that the whole body sags. If the knees won't come off the ground naturally in the curve, don't force them; they will lift after some practice. It is possible that the hands may need to be placed lower down the body, depending on the physique of the student. A little experimentation and some practice will help.

7 Hold the pose for up to one minute, breathing deeply.

8 Bend the elbows slowly to return to position in (1).

Relax and repeat three times in all.

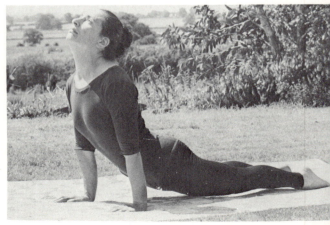

Urdhva Mukha Svanasana: the Dog, both stages

DHANURASANA: THE BOW

In this pose the body looks, in profile, like a bow, the arms being used as a bowstring to draw the feet up. This can help those with slipped discs. It strengthens the spinal cord and acts as a tonic to the thyroid gland, the kidneys, liver and thymus.

Warning: this exercise must not be attempted by people suffering from over-active thyroid glands or from excessive growth of any other ductless gland.

1 Lie face down, flat on the floor.

2 Exhale and bend the knees.

3 Stretch back both arms and grasp the respective ankle (*do not grasp the toes as this could dislocate the foot*).

4 Inhale and at the same time pull the ankles up towards the ceiling (*not towards the head*), keeping the arms stiff, elbows unbent.

5 At the same time raise the chest from the floor and throw back the head as far as possible, looking towards the ceiling. Only the navel area should remain on the floor, the pelvis and ribs being raised so that the body looks like a bow with the arms being the string. When the position is held, the knees should be wide apart for greater ease but as the proficiency increases, the knees and ankles and thighs should be brought closer together. A rocking movement back and forth on the navel should be attempted.

6 Hold the pose for up to one minute.

7 Exhale and slowly relax the limbs returning to the position at (1).

Relax.

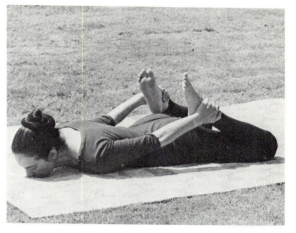

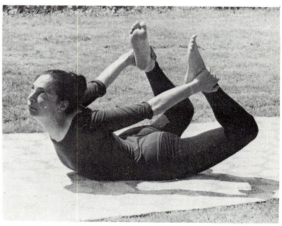

Dhanurasana: the Bow, both stages

ARDHA MATSYENDRASANA: THE SEMI-TWIST

This is one of the few exercises in twisting the spine and can correct certain spinal deformities. It also helps the entire nervous system, the liver, pancreas and spleen and has a pronounced beneficial effect on the kidneys.

First stage

1 Sit erect with legs outstretched in front, arms outstretched at sides and fingertips touching the floor.

2 Slowly turn the whole trunk towards the

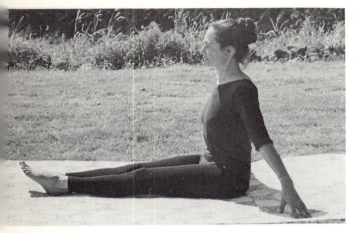

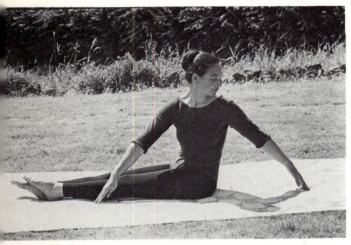

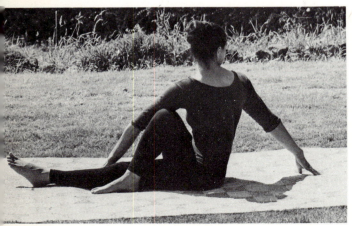

Ardha Matsyendrasana: the Semi-Twist, successive stages

right, looking over the right shoulder with the fingertips of the right hand resting on the floor about 2ft behind the right hip in line with it. The fingertips of the left hand should be touching the floor on the outer edge of the right knee. The head should be turned round as far as possible.

3 Slowly return to the position at (1).

Pause, and repeat turning in opposite direction.

Second stage

1 Sit erect with legs outstretched in front, arms outstretched at sides with fingertips touching the floor.

2 Bend the right knee and place the right foot over the left leg, resting the sole of the right foot on the floor parallel with the left leg, the foot level with the left knee.

3 Exhale and turn to the right, arms outstretched. Pass the left arm, stiff, over the right knee so that the upper arm pushes against the outer side of the right knee. The fingertips of the right hand rest on the floor about 2ft behind the right hip and in line with it. The head is looking as far as possible over the right shoulder.

4 Hold the pose for a few seconds, breathing normally.

5 Slowly face forward and return to position as in (2).

6 Return to (1).

Pause and repeat with the left leg.

Third stage: the final twist

1 Sit erect with legs outstretched in front, arms outstretched at sides with fingertips touching the floor.

2 Raise the right leg, knee bent, until the foot is flat on the floor parallel and level with the left calf.

3 Put the right hand under the right knee and grasp the left ankle, bending the left knee.

4 Draw the left foot and leg under the right knee, pulling the foot as far back as possible, so that the weight of the body is shifted to the left buttock.

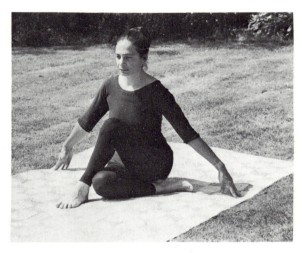

(Do not sit on the left heel — place it close to the right buttock but not beneath it.)

5 Draw the right foot in so that the heel rests on the outside of the lower left thigh, just above the knee, the foot pointing forwards, the knee erect directly below the chin.

6 Stretch arms sideways until the fingertips rest lightly on the floor *making sure that the left knee remains flat on the floor throughout.*

7 Twist the body to the right, arms remaining outstretched and making sure that the outside of the left elbow is on the outside of the right knee.

8 Now with the left hand grasp the right ankle, the left arm being parallel with the right shin.

9 Bend the right arm and lay the back of the hand behind the back of the waist until the fingertips touch the right knee. The head should be turned as far to the right as possible.

10 Hold for up to one minute.

11 Slowly return to the position in (6).

12 After a pause, slowly return to the position in (1).

Pause, and repeat with the opposite side.

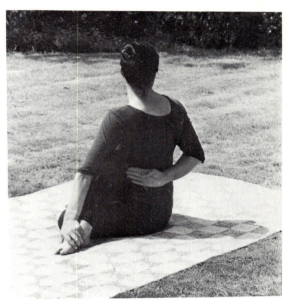

The final twist

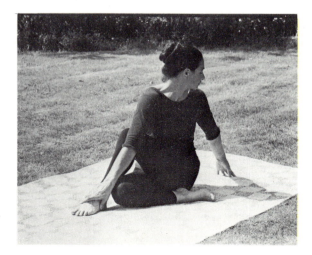

UTTHITA TRIKONASANA: THE TRIANGLE

This exercise has the effect of hastening the removal of toxins from the body. It corrects defects in the legs and develops the chest.

1 Stand erect, feet touching along their whole length, arms by the sides.

2 Place the feet about $3\frac{1}{2}$ft apart.

3 Exhale and point the right foot towards the right and the left foot slightly towards the right.

4 Inhale and raise the arms outwards to shoulder level, keeping elbows stiff and the arms in direct line with the shoulders, palms downwards.

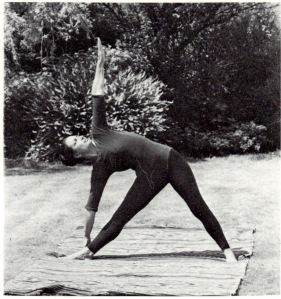

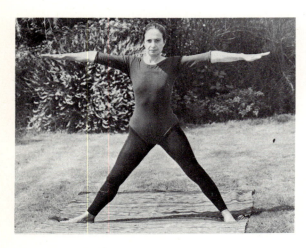

Utthita Trikonasana: the Triangle, both stages

5 Exhale and lower the trunk sideways to the right, taking care not to bend the body forwards, and keeping both arms in a straight line with the shoulders until the fingers touch the floor directly behind the right foot. (At first go as far as possible, but on no account bend forwards.)

6 Turn the head to the left and look along the left arm, keeping the nose parallel to the left arm. Resist the tendency to twist the left hip forward. Both knees must be kept absolutely stiff.

7 Hold the pose for up to one minute.

8 While inhaling, slowly return to the position at (4).

9 Slowly return to the position at (1).

Pause and repeat in the opposite direction.

PARIVRTTA TRIKONASANA: THE REVOLVING TRIANGLE

1 Stand erect, feet touching along their whole length, arms by the sides.

2 Place the feet about $3\frac{1}{2}$ft apart.

3 Exhale and point the right foot towards the right and the left foot slightly towards the right.

4 Turn the upper trunk as far as possible to the right until you are facing backwards, keeping the arms in a straight line level with the shoulders throughout.

5 Bend the trunk down towards the right leg, placing the left hand flat on the floor behind the right foot.

6 Turn the head and gaze upwards along the outstretched right arm. Make sure that you do not lean forwards. Initially it may help to perform this exercise facing a wall to correct any tendency to lean either forwards or backwards.

7 Slowly come upright to position at (4).

8 Slowly return to position at (1).

Pause and repeat in the opposite direction.

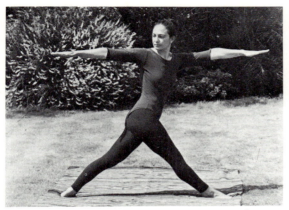
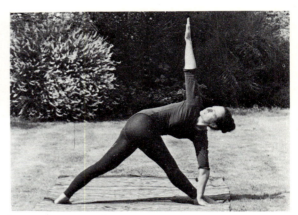

Parivrtta Trikonasana: the Revolving Triangle

UTTHITA PARSVAKONASANA:
THE KNEE-BEND TRIANGLE

As well as providing benefit in the ways of the previous Triangle poses, this helps to relieve sciatica and arthritic pains.

1 Stand erect, feet touching along their whole length, arms by the sides.

2 Place the feet between 4-4½ft apart and at the same time raise the arms sideways to a level with the shoulders, palms facing downwards.

3 Turn the right foot towards the right and the left foot slightly towards the right, keeping the left leg tightly stretched. Bend the right knee until the upper thigh is parallel with the ground and makes a right angle with the calf.

4 Exhale and bend to the right, placing the right palm on the floor behind the right foot.

5 Bring the left arm over the head, keeping the elbow stiff against the left ear and pointing the arm so that there is a continuous stretch from the left foot along the left side to the tip of the left fingers. Turn the head so that it faces upwards.

6 Slowly return to the position at (4).

7 Slowly return to the position at (3).

8 Slowly return to the position at (1).

Pause for a few moments and repeat in the opposite direction.

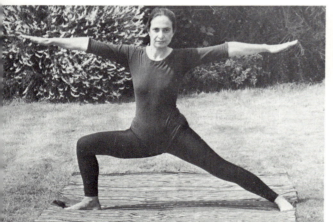
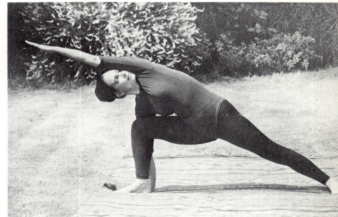

Utthita Parsvakonasana: Knee-bend Triangle, both stages

PARIVRTTA PARSVAKONASANA: THE REVOLVING KNEE-BEND TRIANGLE

This is a more intensified version of the previous asana and helps elimination from the colon.

1 Stand erect, feet touching along their whole length, arms by the sides.

2 Place the feet between 4–4½ft apart and at the same time raise the arms sideways to a level with the shoulders, palms facing downwards.

3 Turn the right foot towards the right and the left foot slightly towards the right, keeping the left leg tightly stretched. Bend the right knee until the upper thigh is parallel with the ground and makes a right angle with the calf.

4 Turn the body to the right until you face backwards.

5 Exhale and bend towards the right leg, placing the left hand flat on the floor behind the right foot.

6 The left arm should be behind the bent right leg so that the right knee fits into the left armpit.

7 Keeping the right arm stiff, move it upwards until it touches the ear and points towards the right so that there is a continuous diagonal stretch from the left leg, through the buttocks and along the right arm. The gaze should be upwards towards the right hand. At all times the left knee should be kept taut.

8 Hold the pose for up to one minute.

9 Slowly reverse the stages until the position at (1) is reached.

Rest for a few moments and repeat in the opposite direction.

ARDHA NAVASANA: THE HALF-BOAT

This strengthens the back and benefits the gall-bladder, liver and spleen.

1 Sit upright on the floor, legs outstretched in front, arms by sides.

2 Clasp fingers together and place them behind the head to cradle the crown.

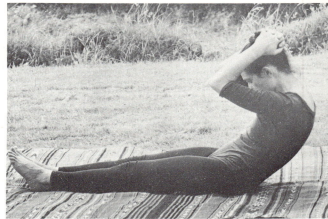

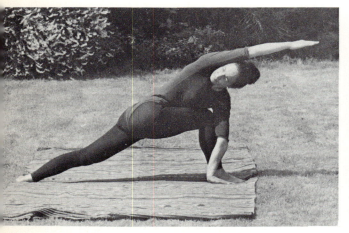

Parivrtta Parsvakonasana:
Revolving Knee-bend Triangle, final stage

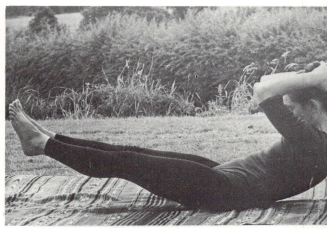

Ardha Navasana: the Half-Boat, both stages

3 Curve the spine and at the same time lean slowly backwards, raising the stiff legs to bring them about 30° from the floor, toes pointing forwards. The head should be at about the same level from the floor as the legs.

4 Hold the pose for a few seconds, but do not hold the breath.

5 Slowly return to the position at (1).

PARIPURNA NAVASANA: THE BOAT

This is beneficial to the intestines.

1 Sit upright on the floor, legs outstretched in front, arms by sides.

2 Arms stiff, by the sides, place palms flat on floor.

3 Keeping the spine rigid, lean backwards and at the same time raise the stiff legs until they make a 60° angle with the floor.

4 The head should be nearer to the floor than the feet.

5 Remove the hands from the floor, stretch the arms in front so that the wrists touch the stiff knees, the back remaining stiff.

6 Hold the pose for a few seconds, breathing gently.

7 Slowly return to the position in (1).

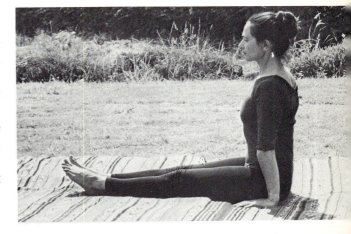

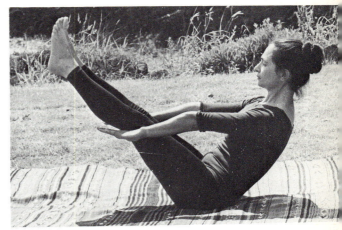

Paripurna Navasana: the Boat, both stages

SIMHASANA: THE LION

First stage

This cures bad breath, relieves a sore throat and helps stammerers.

1 Kneel on the floor making sure that the buttocks are on the floor and the heels touching the thighs, the calves resting on the floor alongside the thighs. If this is impossible, practise daily until the pelvis is more flexible.

2 Stretch the arms out in front and place the extended fingertips on the floor so that the heel of the hand rests on the knees. Elbows must remain stiff.

3 Press the chin against the chest.

4 Stick the tongue as far out and as far down as possible.

5 Cross the eyes and look up.

6 Knit the brows.

7 Stretch the fingers and tense the whole arm and chest and head.

8 Gradually return to the position in (1).

Relax and repeat three times.

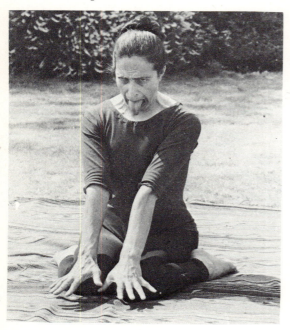

Simhasana: the Lion, first position

Second stage

1 Sit in the Lotus pose.

2 Lean forward. Place palms on the floor and push forward until the weight is on the hands and knees. Now walk forward on the hands so that the spine sags.

3 Press the chin on the chest.

4 Stick the tongue as far down and as far out as it will go.

5 Cross the eyes and look up.

6 Knit the brows.

7 Hold for a few seconds.

8 Slowly walk back on the hands to the position at (2).

9 Slowly return to position at (1).

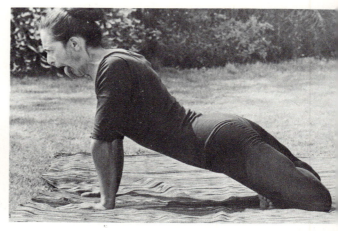

Simhasana: the Lion, second position

PADMASANA: THE LOTUS

Perhaps the most useful, and certainly the best known, of Yoga poses. It is used for meditation and the Buddha is often depicted in it. It cures stiffness in the knees and ankles and once it is mastered, it is an extremely comfortable and stable posture.

1 Sit erect with both legs outstretched in front.

2 With both hands, place the left foot on top of the right thigh well into the groin.

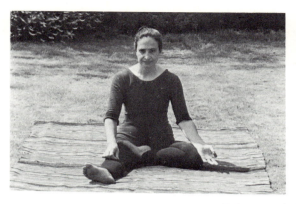 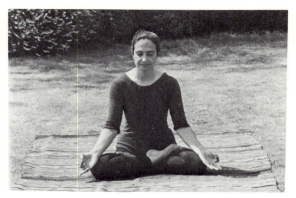

Padmasana: the Lotus, both stages

3 Place the right foot over the left thigh into the groin.

4 The knees must be kept close to the floor.

5 Place the fingers in Jnana Mudra position: first fingers touching the tips of the thumbs, the backs of the hands resting on the knees. *All Pranayama should be done in this position when possible.* Hold for as long as possible. Repeat with feet reversed.

TOLASANA: THE SCALES

This exercise strengthens the wrists, hands and abdomen.

1 Sit in the Lotus pose.

2 Place hands, palms down, beside the body.

3 Bend shoulders slightly forwards.

4 Press on hands until body is raised from the ground, the hands taking the weight.

5 Hold pose for up to five minutes.

Pause and repeat three times.

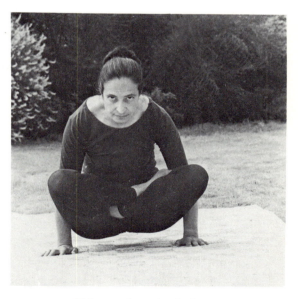

Tolasana: the Scales, final position

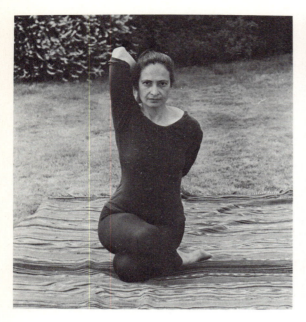 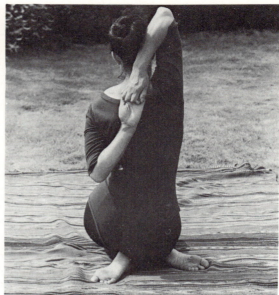

Gomukhasana: the Cow, front and back view of final stage

GOMUKHASANA: THE COW

This exercise cures cramp in the legs, makes the shoulders more flexible and helps relieve fibrositis and varicose veins.

1 Sit erect, legs outstretched in front.

2 Bend the right leg, right foot flat on the floor, knee facing upwards.

3 Thread the left foot through and sit on the left heel.

4 With the left hand, grasp the right ankle, pull it until the right heel is pressed against the left thigh so that the right foot is steadying the balance.

5 Put the right arm back and under so that the back of the arm and hand is pressed against the spine, the fingers pointing upwards.

6 Put the left arm up, bend over the left shoulder and grasp the right fingers, making sure that the left elbow is pointing upwards and that the upper arm is vertical. The head must stay erect, looking forwards.

7 Slowly return to the position in (1).

Pause and reverse the posture.

SIRSASANA: THE HEAD STAND

This pose is believed to rejuvenate the brain, improve the memory and cure insomnia, and relieves colds and coughs.

Warning: this should not be attempted by those with high blood pressure, *nor by women during menstruation.*

First stage: pose 1

1 Kneel down with the buttocks resting on the heels.

2 Place palms of hands flat on the floor, the heel of the hands touching the knees.

3 Put the forehead on the floor, making sure that the buttocks remain on the heels.

4 Turn toes under and shift the weight to the knees.

5 Push the legs straight so that the weight is divided between the head and the toes.

6 Take tiny steps towards the face, bending the knees and widening them until the knees actually sit on the elbows.

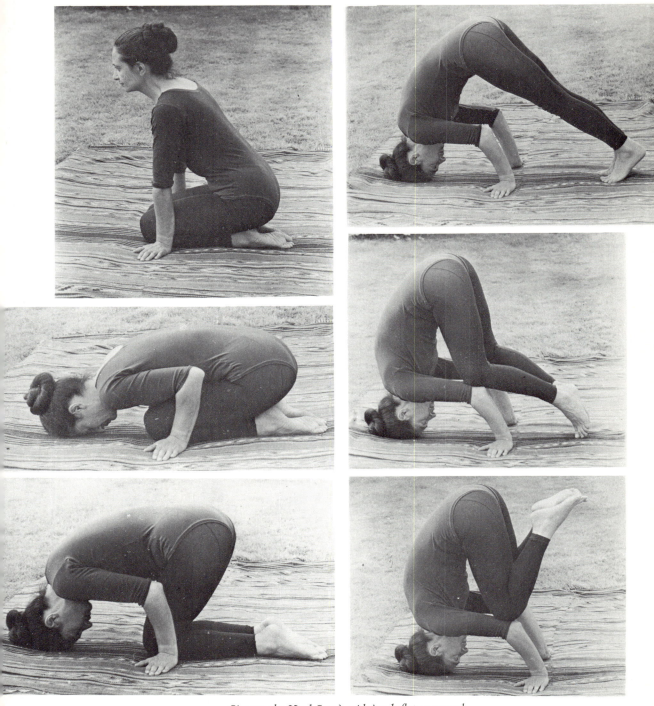

Sirsana: the Head Stand, with hands flat on ground

7 Slowly lift the feet with the knees well bent.

8 Hold pose a few moments and slowly return to position in (3).

9 Hold pose for a few moments before returning to position (1).

Attempt no further head stand exercises until this is perfect and comfortable.

Second stage: pose 1

Repeat as in the previous asana to position in (8).

9 Push down on the hands and slowly straighten the legs until they are vertical, the body in a straight line, stomach held in.

10 Hold the pose for a few seconds, increasing to five or ten minutes.

Warning: there is a strong strain on the neck in this pose and it is advisable to perfect it in the corner of a room where two walls at right angles will support the body should it lose balance. In addition, because of the compression of the neck, it should always be followed by the performance of the shoulder stand which releases the pressure on the spine, especially the neck.

Pose 2

1 Kneel down with the buttocks resting on the heels.

2 Firmly clasp the hands and place on the floor.

3 Put the top of the head (supported by the clasped hands) on the floor.

4 Let the lower arms lie on the floor, the elbows no wider apart than the actual shoulder sockets.

5 Raise the lower trunk, with toes turned under.

6 Straighten the knees, making a V-shape of the body.

7 Walk on tiptoe until the spine is straight.

8 Take a very slight bounce so that the knees come in to the chest.

9 Gradually straighten the legs until they are vertical, making a straight line with the spine, the toes pointing upwards.

10 Hold the pose for a few moments.

11 Slowly return to the position in (8) and then (1).

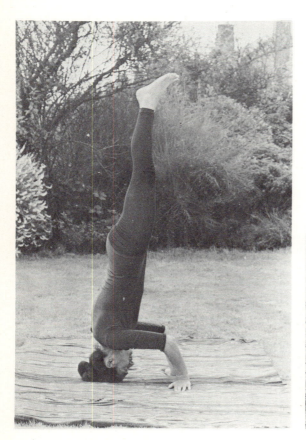

Sirsana: the Head Stand, with hands flat on the ground

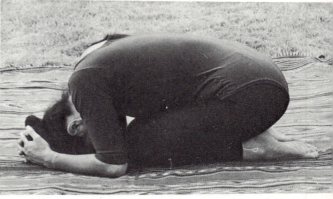

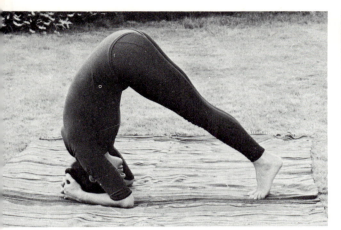
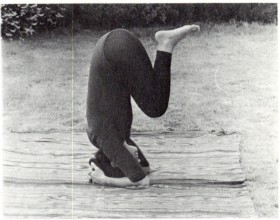

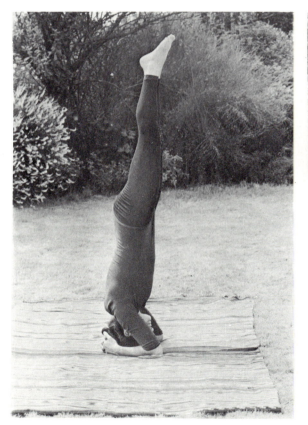
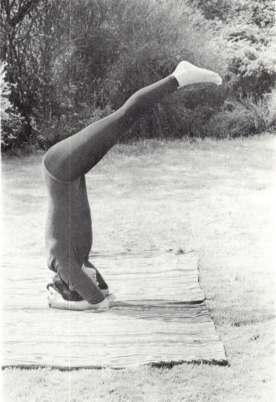

Sirsana: the Head Stand, with hands clasped

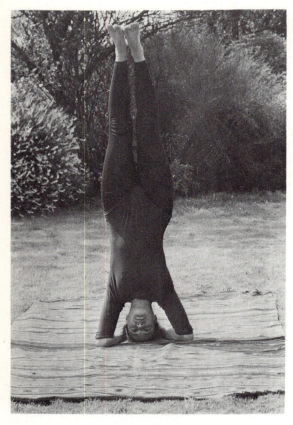

Sirsana: The Head Stand, with hands clasped

When this exercise has been mastered, a variation is to keep the legs stiff going up and coming down (see illustrations).

EYE EXERCISE 1

1 Sit in the Lotus pose, or cross-legged.

2 Hold the index finger of the right hand about 1ft in front of the body as far to the right as the eye can focus on it.

3 Keeping the head facing directly frontwards, so that only the eyeballs move, follow the finger as it moves from the extreme right to the extreme left until it disappears from vision.

4 Move the finger from right to left as in (3).
Repeat three times.

EYE EXERCISE 2

1 Sit in the Lotus pose, or cross-legged.

2 Hold the index finger of the right hand as high above the head as the eyes can focus on it, the head remaining erect and facing forwards.

3 Very slowly move the finger down, keeping it central to the face and follow with the eyeballs until it is as low as the eyes can see it. Make sure that the head does not move.

4 Now move the finger up until it goes out of focus.
Repeat three times.

EYE EXERCISE 3

1 Sit in the Lotus pose or cross-legged.

2 Move the index finger of the right hand in a clockwise direction about 1ft in front of the face.

3 Follow the finger with the eyes, keeping the head facing forwards and perfectly still.

4 Repeat the movement sending the finger anti-clockwise.
Repeat three times.

EYE EXERCISE 4

1 Sit in the Lotus pose or cross-legged.

2 Stretch out the index finger of the right hand right in front of the eyes.

3 Slowly move the finger towards the bridge of the nose, keeping the eyes focused on it.

4 Bring the finger right up to the nose so that the eyes may actually have to cross to see it.

5 Now slowly move the finger away until the arm is extended.
Repeat three times.

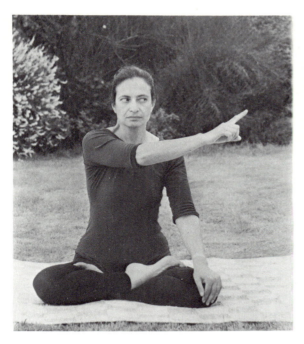

First Eye Exercise

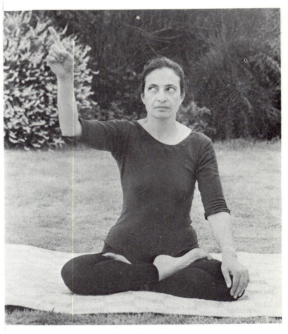

Third Eye Exercise

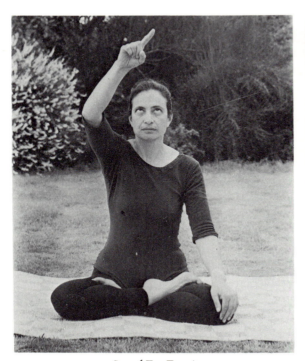

Second Eye Exercise

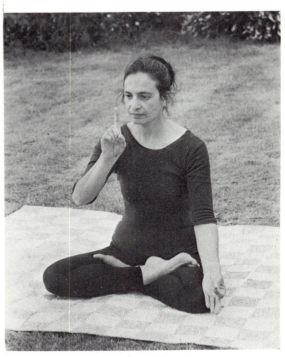

Fourth Eye Exercise

EYE EXERCISE 5: PALMING

In between the three repetitions of eye exercises, the eyeballs should be rested.

1 Sit cross-legged, knees raised.

2 Cup both the palms and place one set of fingers over the other, elbows on knees.

3 Place the palms gently over the eyes so that the eyeballs are in the hollows of the palms and not even the eyelashes touch the hands. *No pressure must be exerted on the eyeballs.*

4 Close the eyes and imagine you are looking at something black.

5 Hold the pose for as long as possible.

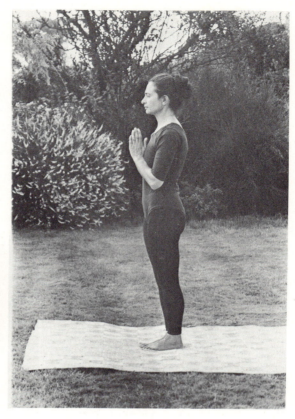

Suryanamaskar: Salutation to the Sun, the beginning position and each of the twelve stages

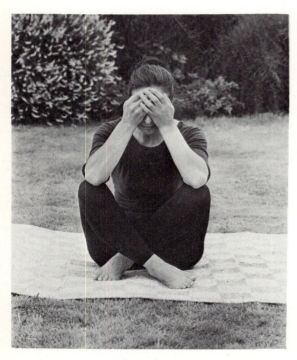

Palming the eyes

SURYANAMASKAR: SALUTATION TO THE SUN

This is a traditional series of asanas which incorporate much of the daily regime in India where many schools lead the children through a series of Yoga exercises each morning. As well as being a symbolic beginning to the day, Suryanamaskar limbers up the muscles, limbs and organs. It should be performed once, twice or three times but slowly and without pause.

1 Stand erect, feet together, palms together just beneath the chin in a gesture of salutation. Exhale.

2 Raise the arms, inhaling at the same time. Part the palms and continue raising arms over the head and slightly backwards, arching the spine.

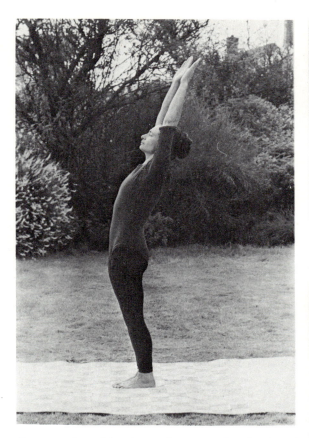

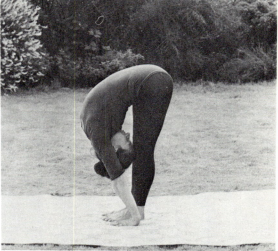

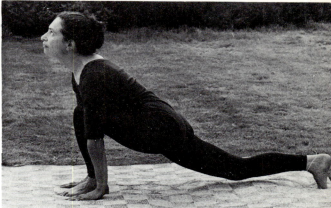

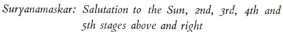

Suryanamaskar: Salutation to the Sun, 2nd, 3rd, 4th and 5th stages above and right

3 Bend down and place the palms on the floor beside each foot, bending the head on the knees. Exhale at the same time.

4 Stretch back the right leg, toes turned under, until the knee is about 1in from the ground and the left leg calf is vertical to the ground, the knee at right angles to the floor. Inhale at the same time. Throw back the head, look upwards and arch the back.

5 Stretch back the left leg parallel to the right, the feet together, making an inverted V-shape of the body. The head should almost touch the ground. Retain the breath.

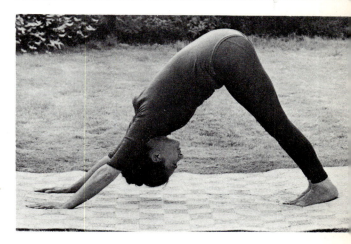

6 Slowly lower the whole body to the floor until every part is touching it except for the pelvis which is just a few inches raised from it. Exhale at the same time.

7 Inhale and putting all the weight on the hands with the elbows stiff, throw back the head and let the body sag so that just the knees, toes and hands are on the ground.

8 Slowly return to the inverted V-position in (5) and hold the breath.

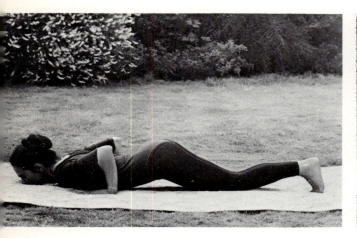
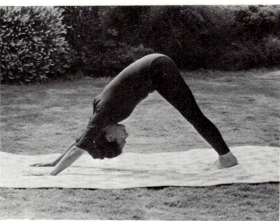

Suryanamaskar: Salutation to the Sun, 6th, 7th, 8th, 9th and 10th stages on this and facing page

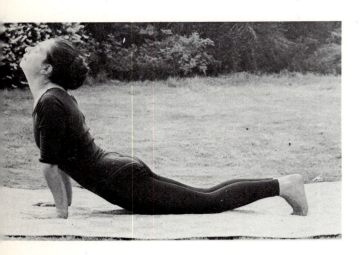

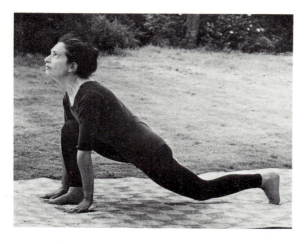

9 Continue holding the breath while lifting the left hip up to bring the left foot forward to a position between both hands as in the position at (4).

10 Exhale and return to the position at (3) with the legs stiff, the trunk bent over and both hands on the floor beside the feet.

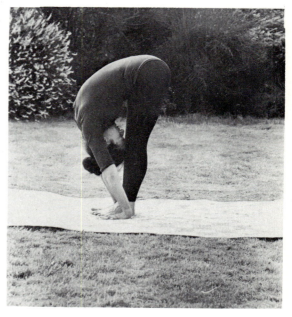

11 Inhale and sweep both arms up straight over the head, arching the back into the position at (2).

12 Exhale and slowly lower the hands, palms together, into the salutation pose of (1).

Repeat with other leg.

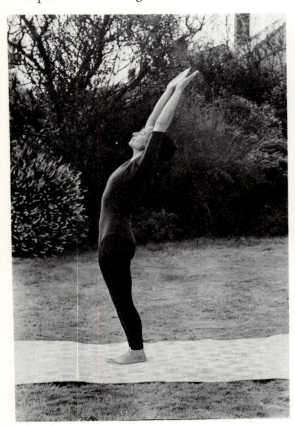
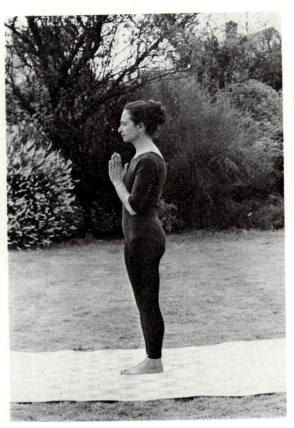

Suryanamaskar; Salutation to the Sun, 11th and 12th stages

13 Concentration

It might be argued that the practice of concentration is, in fact, no part of Hatha Yoga. On the other hand students who practise both agree that concentration helps them to maintain the more advanced poses. Conversely the performance of each asana teaches concentration because it is essential to be aware of the body's every movement if the asana is to be performed correctly and diligent attention is necessary to maintain the pose precisely. Thus if no other specific exercise in concentration was performed, the powers of concentration would be increased and developed solely by the practice of Hatha Yoga. This, of course, presupposes that the student obeys the instructions to perform the asanas using his mind as well as his body.

In any case, no single Yoga path is entirely separate from the others. They overlap and intermingle repeatedly and since the aim of Yoga is to improve the quality of life, it follows that whatever practice aids progress it should be followed. But why concentration? And, more to the point, how can it be developed? The benefits are multiple and well known by those fortunate few who can concentrate without effort. The rest of us, however, can benefit enormously if we follow certain directives.

The main advantages of increased concentration are as follows:

1 To increase our powers of observation. Most people can spend hours in a room and come out unable to answer the most general questions about it. Where was the light switch? What colour was the carpet? How many pictures were there? Similarly most people are unable to describe the clothes worn by someone with whom they have spent the past evening.

Perhaps none of these trivial details matter. But supposing they did? Supposing it was suddenly imperative to recall exact observations of the previous day? Very few would be able to remember, because while our eyes may pass over objects, the details are seldom registered on the brain. The attention is wandering like a butterfly flitting from flower to flower. You actually see, but do not allow the brain to take in the images to reinforce the impression. The mind is unfocused and rather like a computer; unless a certain point is deliberately fed into it, that point cannot be recorded and stored.

2 Concentration strengthens the memory. If the eyes deliberately light on an object and note its colour, shape and size and the brain pays full attention to the sense being used, it will usually comply and store the details. Then, when tapped, the trained memory will obligingly disgorge its contents. This is particularly useful for students who find difficulty in recalling what they have read.

One primary exercise which helps is for the beginner to make notes of whatever he reads. It could be a novel, a newspaper article or a poem. It doesn't matter if he never again looks at his notes; the fact that he has crystallised his impressions and thoughts sufficiently to set them down on paper is enough to have registered them in his memory. It is a small, simple exercise, but one of the most effective.

Yoga philosophy is essentially practical and its insistence on living in the present moment affirms this policy. Those who dwell on the past or continually anticipate the future cannot fully apply their energy to the present moment. The student, therefore, should always try to focus his mind on the matter in hand and let the past and future look after themselves. Of course one must learn from the past and prepare for the future, but not when the mind should be attending to the immediate present.

In this way the person is at peace with himself. He can spend his energies, both mental and physical on the work of the moment, knowing that the rest will be given due consideration afterwards. Concentration is, in fact, like a time-and-motion study of thought. There is an economy of emotion, and superfluous mental energy is reduced to a minimum.

3 Yoga concentration brings peace of mind, for when the brain is focused on one thing at a time, the person is not fragmented and harassed. He can apply himself fully to the immediate task, cutting out distractions so common in the unruly thought processes. It is a kind of liberation known only to those who have tried it and it brings many benefits. By such single-minded concentration, more work is done in a much shorter time. Many people protest that they have not enough time to practice Yoga daily but in fact they would have enough time and even some to spare if they learnt how to concentrate, for they would achieve greater efficiency and would accomplish more in a shorter time.

4 Yoga concentration opposes the waste of energy, whether physical or mental, and nothing wastes energy quite so much as being frustrated. Visualise the situation where you are prevented from doing something you wish to do. Imagine what it feels like having to ignore your own desires because you must comply with your obligations. There is frustration and resentment. But when you have trained your mind to concentrate literally on the present moment, the current task, the problems and dilemmas resolve themselves. The mind, so to speak, wears efficient blinkers and obeys your instructions. You are the master of yourself. This is an essential part of Yoga.

Concentration is impeded by tension. Imagine trying to ride a bicycle with the muscles rigid and the body unbending. Balance would be impossible and most likely you would fall off. But if you could be reasonably relaxed, you would be able to bend the body to correct the wobbling. Similarly with the mind. If you can, like bamboos, bow before the wind, that is, if you are quite prepared for either success or failure, the chances are that you will maintain mental equilibrium whatever life brings.

Since the idea of Yoga is to gain control over both body and mind, and we accept that a restless mind means a restless body, the following exercises are asanas of the mind. So that if the entity is tackled from both ends, mind and body, successful control of both will be the result. To begin with they can be practised at any time. It need not be in the solitude of the Yoga exercises, nor in the period of relaxation. You can start at the bus stop, on a railway station or at the breakfast table, so long as you can keep your full attention on the practice.

EXERCISE I

Since most people have a better visual than aural memory, and abstractions are more difficult, it is best to start with a flower, a plant, a leaf — preferably something pleasing to the eye. If you are indoors, place the object to be studied on a stool or a table at eye level: do not hold it or the sense of touch will complicate the mental processes. If outdoors, choose an object *in situ* — perhaps a growing plant or clump of grass. Indoors, sit cross-legged and, without-staring hard or knitting the brows, slowly and deliberately examine the object but do not turn it round. At this stage you are only interested in the side facing you. Notice the shape of its parts: in the case of a flower, the leaves, petals, stem and so on. Observe the colours and how the shades vary from part to part. Observe the texture and the overall shape. If it has a pronounced perfume, note that, too. After about thirty seconds, close the eyes and try to project the image on the mind's eye. Most people find it impossible at first. Even without achieving a mental picture, they are unable to answer their own questions about the leaf formation or just where there are different shades of colour.

Now open the eyes and have another look at the object, particularly noticing those parts which eluded the memory with the eyes shut. Repeat this procedure for about one minute. To extend it further defeats the object of the exercise, for it is easy to become weary of precise examination until the mind has been limbered up. Don't discard the object, but put it to one side. If it is indoors and if it is a cut flower, put it in water and return to look at it during the day. Meanwhile try to explain and describe it, to a child if there is one around, or even aloud to yourself. Try to draw it or to write a few descriptive lines about it, and whenever you are unsure of one of the details, go and have another look at it.

Each day try to increase the time spent in observing the same object, from one minute to two. As the picture of it begins to build up in the mind, you can try looking at it from another angle, so that within a few days every facet of the object should be familiar to you. Later in the week, try to list every single fact that you can remember about it, bearing in mind that if it is a living object it will probably change a little every day. A flower's petals may open or even fall; its leaves may shrivel or change colour. But the daily practice will sharpen the memory and the powers of observation, and in about one week the mind will have stored every detail of it and of its gradual changes. Only then has the exercise come to an end and the object can be discarded.

Now try the same exercise with a different object. For busy people who cannot spare the time to perform the exercise at leisure, the object might be a tree, perhaps outside an office window. For town dwellers or those with irregular working habits, it could be the salt pot on the breakfast table. Most Yogis advocate a natural, organic object whenever possible but as the purpose of this exercise is to train the mind, it doesn't matter too much if the only suitable object for study is man-made. The method of concentration is just the same; regular study followed by seconds when the eyes are closed and the image projected on the mind's eye. The object is only exchanged for another when its details are firmly entrenched in the mind.

It must always be remembered that if, as often happens, stray thoughts cross the mind during the concentration exercises, they must not be forced out. They must be received, considered for a second or two, and then 'told' that they will be considered more fully at a more appropriate time. In this way no force is used. Should you try to push them away, these extraneous thoughts tend to return repeatedly at frequent intervals or else retreat into the subconscious where they might manifest themselves in dreams or fantasies. As the concentration exercises continue far greater control over one's thoughts is rapidly developed, and so it is usually only the beginner who has to cope with mental intrusions.

It might be argued that this kind of concentration is unnatural, and so it is. But in today's civilisation who can say what is natural and what is not? Much of our life-style is unnatural. We live in predetermined homes, we follow predetermined rules. We obey conventions that were never determined by nature but as this is the only kind of living we know, there is little we can do about it. Yoga, it might be said, is to liberate us from the worst aspects of civilisation. It aims to give us free will, to train our body and mind to serve ourselves and no one else. For in the modern world, only by achieving our own potential can we hope to serve humanity and to improve ourselves.

EXERCISE 2

Begin by thinking of a symbol — a tree, a horse, a waterfall and so on. For example, if the chosen symbol is a tree, draw a diagram with a skeleton tree in the centre and draw short lines radiating from it to perimeter, like rays from the sun. At the end of each line write the name of something directly appertaining to the tree — a twig, leaf, flower, bird or nest — but do not let the mind take a further step and visualise, say, a bird flying as all the objects must relate *directly* to the tree. The rays are radiating *inwards*, not outwards. As soon as the mind seizes an object relating to the tree, the mind must return to the tree; it must not move on to second links, say a caterpillar or a butterfly. Keep this process up for about five minutes or until the supply of direct links has become exhausted.

If the symbol chosen is say, a waterfall, the radiating lines could lead to pebbles, stream, river and estuary, and between times it could take in river banks, their vegetation, frogs, trout, rats and so on.

The aim of this exercise is to concentrate the mind on the centre point while still remembering the perimeter and relating it to the centre without wandering off to associated objects indirectly linked with it. This exercise should be performed, a week at a time, using several symbols until the brain is trained to follow one distinct line of thought of an object with its immediate periphery.

EXERCISE 3

This is to increase the powers of imagination. Imagine an acorn. Sit cross-legged, if possible, and close the eyes. If by this time the brain is sufficiently well trained to cope with the concentration exercises without strain, they can be performed during the Yoga periods of relaxation. Some people, however, find this impossible and find their bodies becoming tense if they try to incorporate the mental exercises while physically relaxing. The exercises, then, can be done at any time of the day.

Take the imaginary acorn and plant it. In the mind's eye see the tiny roots form. See the first shoots appear and the first leaves unfold. Twig by twig, branch by branch, see the superstructure develop. Leaf by leaf, flower by flower, watch it develop into a fully grown tree. Now, with its basic shape clear in the mind, observe it throughout each season; in full summer foliage with the sun playing on it and the deep shade beneath. In autumn when the leaves change colour, curl and start to fall. In winter when the branches are bare and their forms outlined with frost or snow. In spring when the buds fatten and it is so difficult to discern the first one to burst. Extend the imagination to include the daffodils beneath as they grow and to the birds beginning to nest in the branches. But do not go beyond the immediate vicinity of the tree; rather regard it as framed by the confines of the mind. Take as much time as possible and go into as much detail as you can.

This exercise can be adapted to the growth of a baby, but, it must be stressed, not to a child loved by the student. Too many emotions and intrusive thoughts might intervene and cause the attention to stray. It is better to consider an imaginary baby, as impersonal to the student as the acorn. The exercise is ended when the student can recall in detail the final image in its full maturity with all his picture-history clearly visual in the mind's eye. As in the earlier exercises, each of the objects associated with the main symbol must be directly linked. It is not to be confused with the 'word association' tests popular with psychiatrists.

EXERCISE 4

This is a development of the previous exercises. Think of an apple. Bite it and imagine the taste and the feel of the teeth penetrating first the skin and then the flesh. Imagine finding a pippin within. Plant it, see its roots forming, the first shoot, the growth of the tree to maturity. See the flowers and later its first fruit. See the apple changing colour from green to red. Pick one, smell it, bite into it and feel the juice run down the chin. Feel the fresh waxiness against the lips. Use all the senses, try to hear the sound of the teeth crunching into the apple. When the apple has been mentally eaten, discover the pippin within so that the exercise has gone full cycle.

This process can take up to half an hour, and the longer the better. It demonstrates that the student is using to the full his powers of observation and imagination. Only when the whole cycle of pictures and sensual impressions are firmly imprinted in the mind should the exercise be concluded.

EXERCISE 5

Instead of using a mental image, take a candle, light it and place it at eye level 2–3ft away. Do not stare at the flame; this is bad for the eyes. Half-close the eyes and look at the lighted candle for several seconds noticing the shape of the flame, the colour and its movement. Close the eyes every few seconds and try to remember your observations. At no time should the eyes be allowed to water or become tired. They should just be allowed to rest, without glaring, on the flame for not more than four or five seconds at a time. Again, if intrusive thoughts cross the mind, they should be gently set aside with the resolve to deal with them fully later on.

EXERCISE 6

This is called the Cocoon. Sit comfortably on the floor with the knees drawn up to the chin and the arms wrapped round both knees. Throw a light blanket over the body as the exercise should be performed in complete darkness. Now, with arms entwined round the body, find a convenient pulse — perhaps the wrist, the inside of an elbow or in the throat. Sit very still and, having found the pulse, concentrate on hearing the beat of the heart. Once it is discovered, breathe deeply to a count of heartbeats. Do not try doing the Yoga Complete Breath — this would be too difficult in such a hunched-up position.

Breathe deeply and rhythmically with no retention of breath. Gradually the pulse will slow down as the deep breathing calms the body. It is a kind of back-to-the-womb pose and gives an immense feeling of tranquillity. It is a feeling of being away from the rest of the world without being isolated, a feeling of privacy but not of exclusion. It should be practised for five minutes at a time to begin with, increasing to ten or fifteen minutes after a week or so.

EXERCISE 7

Sit cross-legged, close the eyes and turn up the eyeballs to look up at the 'third eye', the Eye of Shiva or eye of wisdom believed to be situated in the centre of the forehead just above the eyebrows (the site, too, of the pineal gland, a small cone-shaped body of unknown function situated behind the third ventricle of the brain). Although the ancients probably had no physiological knowledge of the brain intricacies, they were always conscious of there being some extra sense behind the fore-head and they pictured it in the shape of a third eye. Most Asiatics have seen representations of it, but those of us who have not should either examine one of the traditional representations or else visualise an ordinary third eye.

This is a classic Yoga exercise and the student should sit relaxed, eyes closed and unstrained, looking upwards and 'seeing' the third eye. At first the closed eyes tend to ache with being turned up. At this point the eyeballs should be lowered, keeping the eyes closed, until the sense of strain disappears and the exercise can then be resumed.

EXERCISE 8

Another classic Yoga exercise, this time of sound. It is particularly suitable for those who enjoy music or who have a keen appreciation of sound. Sit cross-legged alone in a quiet room, close the eyes and intone aloud the word 'om' (pronounced 'awm'). Keep the sound reverberating so that it rises slowly from the chest into the larynx, passes the throat, resounds on the palate and through the nasal passages. It is a symbolic Yoga sound representing all creation — the perfect sound, in fact. Europeans who may find it less symbolic may try another full sound which symbolises one of their ideals. It should be a simple, one-syllable sound for preference, with some resonant consonant.

The aim is to fill yourself with sound so that other thoughts and senses are excluded, as if you were a glass to be filled with water so that air is completely displaced. It would be ineffective to use a musical sound which would evoke memories or images. A pure, single sound is better, no matter which. Although the exercise seems simple, it often takes weeks before it is successful.

EXERCISE 9

This is a little different from the previous exercises since it actually prevents stray thoughts entering the mind. Sit cross-legged, close the eyes and put a forefinger inside each ear. *No pressure must be used or the eardrums might be damaged and fingernails should be cut short and be scrupulously clean.* Inhale deeply and, aloud, make a buzzing z-z-z-z-z sound until all the breath is expelled. Without pause, inhale deeply again and continue the buzzing sound. The whole body seems to be enveloped in the sound and its vibrations.

Having tried all the exercises, the student should experience considerable improvement in his powers of concentration and of memory, but it must be understood that some of them may take years to perfect. To track his progress in each exercise, the student is advised to keep note of the number of times that unwelcome thoughts intrude. He can do this by lowering one finger each time this happens, then at the end of the exercise session he will readily see from the number of fingers he has lowered how often his concentration has been interrupted.

Students are advised to choose the concentration exercises they find easiest and most pleasant, and to practise these regularly. In this chapter they are not arranged in order of difficulty but each one must be tried before a selection is made: it is quite common for a beginner to find one of the more advanced concentration exercises easier than the simplest. It is purely a matter of personal selection, and once a choice has been made, the rest can be disregarded. In this way the student will be able to train his mind and his memory and, ultimately, find he can perform the Yoga asanas with greater ease.

In classic Yoga practice, it is necessary to perfect concentration before attempting meditation (see 'Dharana', Chapter 6). Many people confuse the two, but the former is pin-pointing the mind on one object and that which is immediately linked with it; the latter concerns reaching the very essence of an object by excluding *all* other thoughts — a far more difficult exercise than is realised. The modern cult of transcendental meditation uses the tool of a mantra — a sacred thought — on which to concentrate. This is but a tool and although traditionally it is believed to set up vibrations which are beneficial to both the chanter and to others (even at great distances to which the experienced Yogi can transmit them) the mantra is a means to an end, the end being Samadhi, self-realisation.

Suggested Daily Regime

Section 1

1 SAVASANA   relaxation (pp 36, 37)
2 SURYANAMASKAR Salutation to the Sun (pp 96–100)
3 TRANQUIL BREATHING EXERCISES (exercises 1–5, pp 51–4)
4 THREE NECK EXERCISES (pp 59–60)
5 PADMASANA   the Lotus (pp 88–9)
6 SIRSASANA AND VARIATIONS   the Head Stand (pp 90–4)
7 SARVANGASANA AND VARIATIONS   the Shoulder Stand (pp 66–8)
8 ARDHA-MATSYENDRASANA   the Semi-Twist (pp 81–3)

At least one from each of the following sections

Section 2: FORWARD-BENDING ASANAS

1 HALASANA   the Plough (pp 68–9)
2 PASCHIMOTTANASANA   stretching, all stages (pp 71–3)
3 PADAHASTASANA   the Stork, both variations (pp 61, 74)

Section 3: BACKWARD-BENDING ASANAS

1 MATSYASANA   the Fish (pp 70–1)
2 BHUJANGASANA   the Cobra (79, 80)
3 URDHVA MUKHA SVANASANA   the Dog (p 80)
4 SALABHASANA   the Locust (pp 78–9)
5 DHANURASANA   the Bow (p 81)

Section 4: STANDING ASANAS

1 UTTHITA TRIKONASANA   the Triangle (p 84)
2 PARIVRTTA TRIKONASANA   the Revolving Triangle (pp 84, 85)
3 UTTHITA PARSVAKONASANA   the Knee-bead Triangle (p 85)
4 PARIVRITTA PARSVAKONASANA   the Revolving Knee-bend Triangle (p 86)
5 TADASANA   the Mountain (p 75)
6 VRKSASANA   the Tree, all three poses (pp 76–8)

Section 5: MISCELLANEOUS ASANAS

1 ARDHA NAVASANA   the Half-boat (pp 86–7)
2 PARIPURNA NAVASANA   the Boat (p 87)
3 SIMHASANA   the Lion, both stages (p 88)
4 GOMUKHASANA   the Cow (p 90)
5 THE FIVE EYE EXERCISES   (pp 94–6)
6 TOLASANA   the Scales (p 89)
7 BADDHA KONASANA   restrained angle posture (pelvic loosening, pp 62–3, 65)
8 REMAINDER OF BREATHING EXERCISES (pp 54–5)

Glossary

AHIMSA   non-violence or positive love of all creation.

APARIGRAHA   non-acquisitiveness or non-greed.

ARDHA MATSYENDRASANA   half-twist position.

ARDHA NAVASANA   half-boat position.

ARJUNA   one of the Pandava brothers in the *Mahabharata* and the hero of the *Bhagavad Gita* who symbolises man in his earthly dilemma.

ARTHA   meaning.

ASANA   posture, the third stage in Raja Yoga.

ASTEYA   non-stealing and non-covetousness.

BADDHA KONASANA   restrained angle posture (pelvic loosening).

Bhagavad Gita   the Divine Song containing the essence of Yoga philosophy, part of the epic *Mahabharata* (see ARJUNA).

BHAKTI (YOGA)   love, devotion and worship.

BRAHMACHARYA   sexual restraint or moderation.

BHUJANGASANA   the Cobra posture.

BUDDHA   the Enlightened One. Name given to the founder of Buddhism.

CHAKRA   literally a wheel or circle. Name of nerve centres through which the power of the KUNDALINI moves.

DANA   charity or gift, in the sense of love.

DHANURASANA   the Bow posture.

DHARMA   ethical law, moral way of life through duty.

DHYANA   meditation, the seventh stage in Raja Yoga.

GOMUKHASANA   the Cow posture.

GURU   spiritual teacher; the word means 'weighty'.

HALASANA   the Plough posture.

HATHA   force, made up of positive 'Ha' and negative 'tha' forces.

HATHA YOGA   the way towards realisation through physical discipline.

ISHVARA-PRANIDHRAHA   study of the scriptures and dedication to God.

ISLAM   religion of the Moslems.

JNANA MUDRA   gesture of hands, index finger and thumb making a circle to symbolise the union of the individual with the universal.

JNANA (YOGA)   knowledge, way towards realisation through self-knowledge.

KAPALABHATI   a Pranayama exercise useful for cleaning sinuses.

KARMA (YOGA)   action, way towards realisation through action.

KRISHNA   an incarnation of God. Central figure of the *Bhagavad Gita* who represents the universal force.

KUMBHAKA   retention (of breath) after inhaling or exhaling.

KUNDALINI   the Coiled One, the force which is latent at the base of the spine and is drawn up through the CHAKRAS until it reaches the head.

Mahabharata   Indian epic composed by Vyasa which includes the *Bhagavad Gita*.

MANTRA   sacred thought or prayer which is repeated.

MATSYASANA   the Fish posture.

NARADA   a celebrated Yogi who features in many Indian stories.

NIRVANA   freedom, or extinction of delusions. The goal of Buddhists.

NIYAMA   conduct towards oneself. Self-discipline. Second stage of Raja Yoga.

OM   a mantra symbolising the Supreme.

PADAHASTASANA   the Stork posture.

PADMASANA   the Lotus posture.

PARIVRTTA TRIKONASANA   the Revolving Triangle posture.

PARIPURNA NAVASANA   the Boat posture.

PARSEES   'people from Persia', followers of the Zoroastrian religion of Ancient Persia who became refugees in India.

PASCHIMOTTANASANA   back-stretching posture.

PRANA   the life force.

PRANAYAMA   control of breath. Fourth stage in Raja Yoga.

PRATYAHARA   'gathering towards', control of the senses. Fifth stage in Raja Yoga.

PARIVRTTA PARSVAKONASANA   revolving knee-bend triangle posture.

PURAKA   inhalation, filling the lungs.

RAMAKRISHNA   1836–86. A great Yogi who founded the Ramakrishna mission which teaches the union of all religions.

RAJA (YOGA)   the Royal Path, a deliberate eightfold path to realisation.

RECHAKA   exhalation, emptying the lungs.

SABDA   sound or vibration

SALABHASANA   the Locust or Grasshopper posture.

SAMADHI   supreme conscious state. The ultimate state reached by the Yogi. The eighth stage of Raja Yoga.

SAMYAMA   the last stages of Raja Yoga—concentration, meditation and absorption.

SANTOSA   contentment.

SARVANGASANA   the Shoulder Stand or Candle.

SATYA   truth.

SAVASANA   the Dead posture (for relaxation).

SHIVA   name of a Hindu god of the Trinity, the Destroyer, the others being Brahma, the Creator and Vishnu, the Preserver.

SIMHASANA   the Lion posture.

SIRSASANA   the Head posture or Head Stand.

SOUCHA   purity.

SUKHA PURVAKA   comfortable Pranayama.

SURYANAMASKAR   Salutation to the Sun.

SVADHARMA   the following of one's own destiny or way of life.

TADASANA   the Mountain posture.

TAPAS   austerity or self-discipline.

TOLASANA   the Scales posture.

UJJAYI   Pranayama exercise when lungs fully expanded.

URDHVA MUKHA SVANASANA   the Dog posture.

UTTHITA PARSVAKONASANA   Knee-bending Triangle posture.

UTTHITA TRIKONASANA   the Triangle posture.

VISHNU   name of a Hindu god, the Preserver in the Trinity.

VIVEKA   discrimination. In Yoga philosophy, between the real and the illusory.

VRKSASANA   the Tree posture.

YAJNA   sacrifice.

YAMA   conduct towards others. First stage of Raja Yoga.

YANG   masculine or positive force in Chinese philosophy.

YIN   feminine or negative force in Chinese philosophy.

YOGA   union or yoke which joins the individual with the universal.

YOGI   one who follows any of the Yoga paths.

Bibliography

'Alain'. *Yoga for Perfect Health*. London: Thorson, 1957

Avyaktananda, Swami. *Yoga in Theory and Practice*. Bath: Vedanta Movement, 1972

Bernard, Theos. *Hatha Yoga*. Arrow Books, 1960

Bhave, Vinobe. *Talks on the Gita*. Kashi: Akil Bharat Sarva Seva Sangh, 1958

Hittelman, Richard L. *Be Young with Yoga*. Thomas, 1963

Isherwood, Christopher (ed). *Vedanta for the Modern Man*. Allen & Unwin, 1952

Iyengar, B. K. S. *Light on Yoga*. Allen & Unwin, 1968

Mishra, Ramurti. *Fundamentals of Yoga*. NY: Julian Press, 1959

Prabhavananda, Swami. *Vedic Religion and Philosophy*. Madras: Sri Ramakrishna Math, 1950

—— and Isherwood, Christopher (trans). *How to Know God: The Yoga Aphorisms of Patanjali*. London: Allen & Unwin, 1960

—— ——. *The Song of God*. Mentor, 1957

—— and Manchester, Frederick (trans). *The Upanishads*. Mentor, 1957

Ramacharaka, Yogi. *Hatha Yoga*. London: Fowler, 1963

——. *Hindu-Yogi: Science of Breath*. London: Fowler, 1964

Shelton, Herbert. *Fasting Can Save Your Life*. Chicago: Natural Hygiene Press, 1964

Spring, Clara and Goss, Madelaine. *Yoga for Today*. Thomas, 1959

Vivekananda, Swami. *Bhakti Yoga*. Calcutta: Advaita Ashram, 1955

——. *Hinduism*. Madras: Sri Ramakrishna Math, 1968

——. *Jnana Yoga*. Calcutta: Advaita Ashram, 1955

——. *Karma Yoga*. Calcutta: Advaita Ashram, 1955

——. *Raja Yoga*. Calcutta: Advaita Ashram, 1955

Wood, Ernest. *Yoga*. Pelican, 1972

Yesudian, Selvarajan and Haich, Elisabeth. *Yoga and Health*. London: Allen & Unwin, 1953

Index